Somatic Therapy

A Holistic Guide for Physical Mental Social Spiritual Health & Performance

(Improving Mental and Physical Symptoms With Proven Strategies)

John Payne

Published By **Darby Connor**

John Payne

Somatic Therapy: A Holistic Guide for Physical Mental Social Spiritual Health & Performance (Improving Mental and Physical Symptoms With Proven Strategies)

ISBN   978-1-998769-47-6

No part of this guidebook shall be reproduced in any form without permission in writing from the publisher except in the case of brief quotations embodied in critical articles or reviews.

Legal & Disclaimer

The information contained in this ebook is not designed to replace or take the place of any form of medicine or professional medical advice. The information in this ebook has been provided for educational & entertainment purposes only.

The information contained in this book has been compiled from sources deemed reliable, and it is accurate to the best of the Author's knowledge; however, the Author cannot guarantee its accuracy and validity and cannot be held liable for any errors or omissions. Changes are periodically made to this book. You must consult your doctor or get professional medical advice before using any of the suggested remedies, techniques, or information in this book.

Table of contents

Chapter 1: Feelings And Emotions That Might Arise During Stages Of Grief

This chapter will be opened with a well-known, millennial phrase that is appropriate for this situation. It is okay to not feel okay. Moving on after loss is difficult. It's important not to compare your progress with others. You must heal in your own time and at your own pace.

Do you know what grief is? Most of the time, the hardest reality we confront after losing someone in our lives isn't really the grief caused by the loss but rather the grief of having no choice but to continue living without them. Grief settles deep in our hearts, making the world uninviting.

In simple terms, grief can be described as an emotional response that we have to the present situation. Our ancestry plays a large part in our emotional wiring. The ability to react to danger was a natural part of our evolution as humans. For example, when faced with a predator-like threat, our ancestors' emotions (in this case fear) allowed them to react by either finding ways to remove the threat from themselves or running away from the threat. This is a simplistic view that doesn't take into account the fact that humans are social animals with a wide range of responses to everything around them. (Simons and 2009). It is because of our emotions that we live and thrive. In this way, grief can be as valid as any other emotion.

Emotions can be described as internal responses. They are expressed through physiological and mental channels. The mental channels correspond to the cognitive terms that are attached to the emotion. These could be anger, love, joy or grief. The responses that the mental channels incite in us is a sign of our physiological dimension. If we are angry, our mental channels may trigger a raised heartbeat, palpitations, and a faster heartbeat. You may feel confused and slow when you're grieving. These are physiological responses to cognitive channels.

Both these dimensions are necessary to talk about emotions. This allows it to be distinguished from regular physical activities that can also make us tired, like a long day at work or a hike up the mountain.

What then, is grief? What is grief? It is a mental channel that is accompanied physiological responses such as pain, exhaustion (numbness), and a decline in interest in life. For some, grief may manifest in other forms, including increased heart rate and confusion or an overwhelming sense of inadequacy. Grief occurs after an immediate loss of someone or something close to the victim. While it does not always have to involve a person, we will try to view it through the lens of a spouse. Loss is something that comes along with us all through our lives. However, not all losses come with grief. These two things are not compatible, since sometimes a loss simply serves as a way to accept the fact that life is moving forward. It is possible that we no longer like cartoons in the same way as when we were younger.

Although it may seem like a loss in what we once loved and is associated with grief, it is not a cause for concern. It's part of the normal process of growing up. The opposite is true when loss affects something that is very important to us, something that our lives are not possible without. In this case, the emotional response we get in the form grief is acute. This can manifest in outward actions such as crying, situational sleepiness, increased appetite or loss of appetite, distasteful for human company or excessive attachment towards work.

If you are experiencing this emotional response, I advise you to let it be and to acknowledge it. This would help you start your journey to healing. Too often, society forces us to believe the things we feel are weakness. This is false. It is better to accept your loss and mourning, and to be open to working with it. If you continue to suppress your grief, you'll reach a stage where you are unable to grieve and will be unable to live a normal life.

Everyone grieves differently. However, each method can be used. Kamille Bauer, a motivational speaker, stated that grief is as individual as a fingerprint. Our reactions are often dependent on many factors such as how close we were with our partner, whether the loss was unexpected or sudden, whether we are financially independent and if we have a large family to support. The pain and intensity of your grief will vary from month to month. However, the intensity and causality of grief are important factors to consider. It should be acknowledged and addressed, not ignored. The reality is that grief does not follow a pattern. One day you may feel a little better and the next you will be miserable. It is possible for your emotions to take over and cause you to feel embarrassed. In some cases, shock can make it impossible to talk coherently. It can make all your efforts seem futile. It could make it seem impossible to do the job, or that it is too difficult. It might be all of these, but it could also include something else. There is no single way to grieve.

The next question is now. How long will your grief continue?

The simple answer is, there is no timeline. It is subjective. The intensity of grief varies from person to person. It can last anywhere from two to ten decades, and it can be very different for each loss. It is possible to recover. You can also live your life without restrictions if you have the right social support and emotional strength. This being said, I advise you not to set a timeline for your journey. Don't tell yourself, "I must get better in the next 2 months", "Grief can be ignored by the weak and I will pretend that it doesn't exist", or, "I must not show the world that I am experiencing grief". Even if you feel the pain for a prolonged period of time, like for years, it is still valid. Your response to the situation is different from the response given by others. Your unique personality will dictate your response. In my own experience, it has been clear to me that people grieve differently. Some grieve in more expressive ways, while some others mourn silently. As such, there is no set time frame within which you should stop grieving. There is no proper way to grieve. Any method that helps to get in touch with your emotions and allows you to access your inner turmoil and headspace at any given moment is valid.

It is important to remember that people often grieve in the same way. Therapy is a way to understand that you aren't alone in your sorrow or despair. Different stages are what everyone will experience when grieving. Dr. Elisabeth Kubler, in her book "On Death and Dying" brought this out. This book was published by Newman in 1969 and provides an overview of the five stages of grief each individual experiences following the death or loss of a loved. We will also explore how grief manifests itself over the years that follow the event. Let's first look at Kubler's stages. The stages are not necessarily arranged chronologically. You might encounter several of them at once, or none at any one time.

Kubler has identified the five stages of denial as anger, bargaining (depression), acceptance (Fletcher and 2020). Denial may include a primary emotion such as shock, and refusing to accept that you could be affected by something so terrible. Contrary to popular belief, denial during grief is not harmful. Instead, it serves as a shield and will protect you from being overwhelmed by emotions. It is possible for your thoughts and feelings to be dominated at this stage by the memories, experiences, and special moments you shared with your loved. As a result, you may feel numb. The shock you have suffered has shaken everything about your life. It has changed everything in a matter of seconds. This stage is where you exist in a type of positive reality, which you prefer to the real thing. This helps you regulate your emotions. It also helps you avoid feeling overwhelmed. In simple terms, it is similar to the way you feel when there is too much work. At this stage you might find yourself withdrawing from social events or minimizing contact with others.

The next stage is anger. Anger may last a lifetime or only for a few hours. It can take many forms, such as crying, anxiety, exhaustion or loneliness. Anger develops when you begin to experience the real world and lose the illusion of the favored universe. You might feel angry about the injustice. But, after all, you shouldn't have to suffer so much pain or sorrow. Life may seem unfair. You might look for the fault in the world, then blame your family members and friends. Individuals may feel abandoned at this time. I advise that you feel your anger. If you don't feel it, it will fester inside you like a wound and eventually lead to emotional breakdown. Anger is an instinctive response. It deserves to be expressed. It will eventually end and you can accept it. It can be viewed as something that is holding you back from the world.

The next step is bargaining. Here you try to reach a deal. If you feel that you are unable or unwilling to accept the loss, then you start to make requests in the deep divide. This stage is a sign of deeper denial. You may feel severe guilt if you are unhappy with the outcome. The common feeling is that you should've tried harder, done more or been there for your spouse. You should not let this stage go untreated. If you're facing this, my advice is to slow down and reflect. You have nothing to do what has happened. Sometimes, the world is harsh. The act of beating yourself up about things you cannot control will not make them any more harsh. Be kind to you.

Depression is often associated closely with grief. This stage may bring you to the realization that your loved is gone. Realization sets in, and the sadness follows. Depressed people will spend long periods of time in bed, refuse to go to work, not want to eat or bathe, not clean the house, and allow life to pass you by. Your mind may be asking questions about the meaning of existence, or what it is to live with so much suffering. You shouldn't deny that you feel sad after the death of someone you loved. Everyone experiences mourning. Depression is the main character.

You should also remember that stage depression should not be confused with clinical depression. Depression during grief is an integral part of the situation and a natural outlet for the loss you have suffered. It will decrease in intensity with time. Although it may occasionally rear its head, it will fade away and you can find reasons to be happy. Without medical treatment, clinical depression is more serious and can cause a patient to feel sluggish and irritable. Both are possible, but they can be confused.

This is an assumption that will change as you grow older. Acceptance will come when you reach this stage. Acceptance doesn't automatically mean that your significant others have passed away. Acceptance does not mean that your life is going on without your partner. This is a stage in which you can accept the fact that your life is as it is right now. While you may feel overwhelmed by sadness for days and feel a hollow feeling in your stomach, it will pass and you will be able make coffee and get on with your life. Grief is a process that changes over time. While it may not feel as raw at the beginning, it will still be there for you for some time. But this doesn't mean that you have to end your life.

Other mental health professionals also have their own ideas about how grieving happens. John Bowlby from the UK, a psychiatrist, developed a framework that focuses on the emotional reverberations and effects of loss. His model was called Kubler–Ross Change Curve. It included seven interconnected stages and not five clearly defined ones as previously described (Casabianca at 202). These stages are:

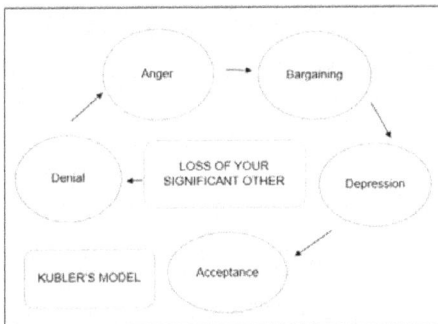

KUBLER'S MODEL

* Shock. This could appear as a sudden, intense, and immobilizing feeling of numbness.

* Denying what has happened and refusing to accept the new circumstances.

* Bliss and anger, as well as a feeling of frustration at the way the world has treated you.

* Depression is a feeling of sadness.

* Experimentation and testing to assess if new changes can fit into existing circumstances.

* This is the stage of decision-making. It includes the first sign that you are optimistic that things will be fine.

* Understanding and integrating new reality, and being ready to face it again (Casabianca; 2021).

Timeframes

I do not believe that you should feel these emotions in a specific time frame. However, the time between the tragedy and the time you experience them will have an impact on the way you handle it. For example, during the first phase, it may seem like your life is a complete rollercoaster. You may even find yourself feeling scattered.

The first year is typically the most difficult. Because you are not only dealing with the emotional consequences of the loss, but also the social and economic manifestations, like the loss of friends or financial support, the first year can be very hard. Birthdays and anniversaries can be especially difficult. It's not necessary to try to solve your grief. You can continue to live in the present and accept it. You need to find a way of using your grief as fuel to your existence. This can be a way to remind yourself of how dear your spouse was to the world, or it may serve as a source for comfort.

You'll have days when your emotions are so intense that you feel like you're going through a nightmare. You may have thought your life was perfect, but now you are a mess of emotions. This is normal behavior. It happens for everyday activities such as when we awaken in the middle of a meal and feel compelled to eat sugary or creamy foods. You can imagine how it can be so hard to keep up with something as simple as a diet. It's enormous. Don't be ashamed to admit that you are feeling more grief than usual. Be present with your emotions and reflect on why you are feeling this way. What song brought back memories of your time with each other? Is it a particular scene from a movie you saw? Is it the way you drank your morning cup of coffee? It could be the smallest thing. This does not mean it is invalid.

People who were initially supportive might become more distant from your grief as time goes by. You will find it difficult to share your grief or how difficult things have been. People rarely like to find themselves in situations where they feel they are being cheated or have done enough. However, this should not be a reason to slow down your grief. Take the time to heal yourself before you decide to get out there and confront the world. Support groups can provide a great outlet for your emotions. Every word you share will affect those who are there. If you're looking to share some of your emotions with others without becoming lonely, a support group for bereavement can be a good place to start. It may also be worth looking for a local organization that supports needlework, cycling, and other hobbies.

Activities that would be easy under normal circumstances, such as lunch out with friends, can seem difficult. It can bring out a lot of anxiety, envy, or a feeling of loss to be around married couples. Even though going out may seem overwhelming, don't feel pressure to do so. Do not go out more than once per week. Inform your loved ones that you might have a late departure or that you are still in recovery.

Don't let anyone decide what you should do next. It's your grief, it's your loss, and it is your time to heal. You may hear others say the worst things, but they might not have the best intentions. This could make you feel insensitive about the impact of their words on your life and the way you should be outside enjoying the sun. Sometimes they may tell you that you should not be grieving. Be aware that these realizations must come to you by yourself and not be forced upon you by others. Give yourself space, love, and time. You can tell others to "move onto" when they ask. You can repeat this several times until you get the point. Always remember that each individual is different in their approach to handling social and personal situations. You might think someone is being cheerful and coping well with life, when in fact they may be more serious than you. Your grief is not a game. Do not place expectations on the validity or length of your grief.

Sometimes, problems occur because we think we are not grieving accordingto the accepted norms of society. We believe there is a correct way to grieve. This happens because we assume that everyone grieves exactly the same. Remind yourself that you do not have to grieve the same as someone else.

Anger may last for one year, while it might take one month for another. This can lead to undue discomfort. You may believe that you should be able get out of this stage sooner. Another option is to channel anger in a different manner, instead of being vocal. Your way of doing business does not have to be wrong. Even if things seem slow, it doesn't mean you should stop being angry, depressed, or scared.

You may not be able to do it all by yourself, however. It could be that you have difficulty focusing on the job. You may be the sole caregiver. However, now you have to deal not only with your own sorrow but also the burden of soothing the pain of a child. You might feel discomfort that is more physical than you realize. You feel drained and unable take your medication or eat. The idea of not having a partner makes it feel unwell. These symptoms can become more intense and persistent if they continue. It is possible to receive tremendous support if your sorrow becomes unbearable and you cannot cope.

Let's first look at a worksheet. This worksheet was inspired in part by "Tasks of Mourning", the handout that draws upon information provided by J. William Worden. The worksheet's purpose is to show that all grief expressions, no matter their intensity or duration, are normal. There are ways you can channel grief and use it for your own good (Worden (2018)).

TASK NUMBER: TASK REQUIREMENT

Task 1 - Accept that loss is an irreversible, real, and tangible event. When you are able to accept the loss at both the physical and emotional levels, this task is complete.

Task 2: Legitimize and accept your grief. A common sign of grief is despair, resentment or remorse. It's easy to reduce difficult feelings by suppressing or avoiding them. Dealing with grief is different. It involves acknowledging and addressing your feelings and critically thinking about them. This is crucial for healing.

Task 3 is Adjustment to The Outer World. It is entirely acceptable to believe that the world will not be the same after the loss of a loved. You should not avoid the outside world and try to ignore it. Instead, you need to make an effort to adapt to the new circumstances. This does not mean that you should abandon your previous existence. You simply need to accept the new one.

There are internal adjustments that can be made. These will help you reshape who you are, especially if there is a crisis in your independence or you cannot see yourself without the deceased.

To survive, you'll need to make adjustments externally. You may need to start a job or learn to manage your finances. These are all strategies that will help you make it through life.

Last but not least, spiritual adjustments might be made through a realignment of your worldview. Accept the feelings of this realignment. Now ask yourself what beliefs and values you're willing to accept.

Task 4: Choose other options to keep the memory of the deceased alive and well. The last task is all about balance. It helps you realize that remembering and honoring someone's memories is not the exact same as stopping your everyday existence because they have passed away. When you are done, you will reach a point of equilibrium between what is and what was.

This worksheet can be returned to as many times as needed. The four tasks are not a one-time assignment. Instead, this worksheet is intended to guide you for as long as your journey takes.

Next, we'll be discussing the physical effects of grief and how they could be affecting us. These sensations are not an indication to panic or stress. Without a loved-one, life can be very difficult.

Chapter 2: Physical Effects Of Grieving And How To Deal With Them

Deep grief can feel like a place, a point on a time map. If you are stuck in the forest of your sorrow, it is hard to imagine how you will ever find your way back to a better place. Sometimes hope is found in someone who can remind you that they too have been there and that they are now better.

- Elizabeth Gilbert, Eat, Pray, Love.

Before we go into the details of how grief can feel like a knife in your chest, I want to say that this isn't a common feeling. I know of people who have talked about the grief they feel, and not just how it affects their bodies. Kristin, a close friend, was afflicted by grief. My friend Kristin used to tell me that just being alive caused her pain. I was initially confused when I first heard this. I was initially confused when I heard this. I continued to research the topic and found surprising results that opened my eyes to new knowledge about how we are all able to sense the signs around us.

Truth is, it's amazing how tangible grief can feel. It is possible for severe grief to cause physical discomfort. Many people mistakenly believe that sorrow is a single emotion. However, natural grief is a strong, complex and sometimes uncontrolled response that human beings experience after a traumatizing or stressful event such as the loss or death of a loved. Suffering can affect us not only mentally, but also cognitively, biologically, and intellectually. Suffering may affect many parts of your body, both physically and emotionally. The neural, nervous, circulatory, and digestive systems are the most commonly affected areas of the body by sorrow. A severe form of sorrow could cause an increase in heart rate, chest discomfort or irregular pulse. Your heart feels pain, and your body may feel tingling. You may feel your stomach clench or your body become cold from merely recollections. When you are in distress your mind will rush, making it difficult for you to fall asleep. This keeps you awake at night, and makes you tired at work.

Research has shown the dramatic effects of grieving on the human body. In a 2014 study in Ageing and Immunity, it was found that those who have lost a close friend or family member may be more at risk for developing infectious diseases. This is especially true in widows and other elderly widows (Vitlic and colleagues, 2014). Cortisol, the stress hormone that causes grief, can be increased which can in turn cause the dysfunction of the human immune system. Cortisol is otherwise balanced by the DHEA (Dehydroepiandrosterone) hormone which is important for the effectiveness of our body's neutrophils (agents that fight against infections). Unfortunately, our DHEA levels drop as we age, especially after we reach thirty. We are more likely to experience the side effects stress has on our bodies. Your immune system attack will make you tired and more susceptible to infections. The pain of losing a loved person can cause high blood pressure and an increase in the chance of blood clots.

Stress is a factor that links the emotional and physical manifestations to grief. The stress that we experience (emotional or physical) can often be absorbed by our bodies. However, the former can also cause neuron damage. Stress can cause more problems if it becomes chronic. Grief can cause inflammation which can worsen existing health issues or lead to the creation of new ones. Acute inflammation is a condition in which there is an injury to the internal system and the body is healing. Chronic inflammation, often caused by stress, is a condition in which there may not be any internal injury. This means that the body is energized and ready to heal. This type of inflammation can result in insulin being reduced, which can lead directly to lifestyle diseases like diabetes. It can also lead blindness, arthritis and cancer. A second study was conducted at Johns Hopkins University (Maryland) and revealed that heart attacks can be caused by acute emotional heartbreak. This was called "broken heart syndrome", and is very similar to the symptoms of cardiac disease.

An increase in grief can lead to a greater need for self-medicating. The most tempting candy can be a bottle of painkillers and over-the–counter sleep medication. These painkillers may temporarily provide relief but long-term, unsupervised use can result in a decline in your body's natural immunity and stress levels. It can reduce the taste of your food, make it less tasty, increase blood pressure and clots, increasing your risk of having a serious heart attack.

While we have given a general overview of how grief can affect our physical health, let's examine each one.

* First, grief can cause increased heart problems. This is due to the cumulative chronic stress that we just described. Sometimes the grief can be so intense that individuals may experience heart attacks,

chest pains, severe shortness and difficulty breathing.

* The second is grief that can manifest through lowered immunity. It can increase the risk of viral infections such influenza.

Another side-effect of grieving is pain and swelling in the joints. This is caused by increased stress-related cortisol levels. They can have a numbing impact on muscular function and, if left untreated long-term, they can lead lifestyle diseases like hypertension, clinical obesity, and type 2 diabetes.

* Unexpressed grief may cause stress to build up in the human digestive system. This can happen naturally, for example, by attracting to "comfort foods" - food with high levels of oil, processed ingredients, and harmful additives. Other signs include an increase in appetite, overeating, emotional eating and irritable intestinal syndrome.

* Unexpressed grief can also have an indirect physical effect. For example, unhealthy

coping mechanisms like using painkillers or alcohol, smoking, or self-harm, may lead to the development and use of harmful coping methods. This can have serious consequences on both your mental and physical health.

* It is possible for people to not acknowledge their grief, which can lead to sleep problems, as well as a desire or need to self-harm due exhaustion. The body has the ability to heal and rebuild itself during sleep. If it is not, then everything can seem twice as confusing and frustrating.

The research cited above is objective. It is not intended to increase stress levels. It is important to remember that these long-term problems are more likely if you don't recognize your grief and allow it to fester within your body. It is easy to keep our suffering a secret and punish ourselves every single day. This can lead to physical trauma. A Circulation journal 2012 study found that individuals' propensity to suffer heart attacks or failures increased twenty-one percent on the day following the death. The same was true for six weeks (Romm, 2014.). This risk could even last for a whole month. We all have heard stories about people dying from grief. This is not a myth. People can die from grief. If you find yourself avoiding events and focusing your energy on negative thoughts, it is possible that you are subconsciously looking for ways you can avoid facing your problems. It is possible that you don't even know you are doing this. Experts suggest that this is a sure-fire way to develop clinical depression. Avoidance is a waste of energy that puts too much strain on your system. It refuses to allow your body's natural systems to understand new realities and take steps toward healing. The clinical consequences of avoidance go beyond depression. It can cause chronic inflammation and weaken the immune system.

My solution: Find a way that you can express your sorrow. My advice? My advice: Somatic Therapy.

Therapy can seem intimidating at first. It is often dismissed as something people with "issues", who turn to it. It's impossible to believe that this could be further from reality. Therapy is a way to get in touch with your inner self. It helps you cope with emotional issues that may not be addressed by pills or alcohol. It allows you to be grounded, to know yourself and your capabilities. While medicine can provide temporary relief for the immediate problem of sleeplessness, therapy will focus on the root cause. If you depend on medications to get you to sleep, there will be a time when you can't get rest. Therapy on the otherhand, helps you discover what is causing you sleeplessness, what is in your subconscious mind, and how to overcome it using your own willpower.

Let's do one thing right now. According to the National Alliance on Mental Health, 1 in 5 Americans have a mental condition. Only 40% seek therapy out of this staggering figure. This can lead you to have more difficult issues in the future, such as difficulty working or supporting your family, increased vulnerability to accidents and health problems, frequent hospitalizations, and grievous self injury (Raypole, 2019). Therapy is crucial in helping you realize how beautiful your life truly is and how you deserve to live happy. Actually, therapy comes from Latin and literally means "healing". This is what we want, even in the face such devastating loss.

So what is Somatic treatment? Somatic therapy originated in the 1970s. It was developed by Dr Peter Levine who is a renowned psychologist with over forty-years of experience in trauma and stressful therapy. Somatic Therapy is a body-oriented form of therapy that examines the interconnectedness between the mind and the body to help release any stress that may have an adverse effect on your psychological and physiological well-being. It means "of body" and is fundamental to understanding the concept. Somatic Therapy, 2002. It is important to seek out treatment that will allow you to heal your mind and restore balance in your body. Somatic therapy uses both psychotherapy and physical therapy to achieve this. This allows you to release stress and heal your trauma-related areas.

Conventional psychotherapy can address a wide variety of mental and psychological health issues. Somatic psychotherapists believe it is possible to address deep personal issues through close monitoring of the body's information flow. The adaptive immune system of a person is affected by past trauma. People who are experiencing behavioral or biological difficulties could also be suffering from hormonal imbalances, digestive issues or friction in specific areas such as the chest or sternum.

Sometimes, our physical and emotional habits can cause us to feel restricted. They are like a tightening of our inner selves. We cannot get out. This can cause anxiety and panic as well as a lack or ability to control your emotions. Somatic therapy helps individuals understand trauma and how it can lead to dysfunction.

They use this awareness to help them navigate their painful thoughts and emotions. The ability to be more conscious of your body over time can lead to a greater awareness and mastery of techniques that can release tension and stress. Mindful meditation, breathing exercises as well awareness of body sensations and grounding techniques are some examples. The therapy response is encouraged to develop new thoughts and behaviors in order to respond better to trauma experiences. Somatic therapy is an effective way to heal those who experience post traumatic stress or anxiety, depression anger, anxiety, addiction and a combination of all of these emotions into one grief.

Somatic therapy focuses on your body's freeze or response. This is similar the body's fight/flight response when there is the perception that something is wrong and you want to get away from it. These physical signs can include increased adrenaline, respiration speed, increased hormone secretion or rapid heartbeats. Your body freezes when it perceives a threat. This happens often after a traumatic event that you cannot escape. It is impossible to run away, so you do the best you can and stop your thoughts and emotions running. This is a huge problem and will stop your healing. Somatic therapy is a holistic approach to helping you deal with trauma in a holistic manner and help you heal.

In the next chapter we will examine different somatic interventions that can help you deal the pain and trauma caused by the loss of a loved. It is possible that you are wondering what to look out for in a therapy.

Look for a therapist who is experienced in somatic therapy. These are your obvious concerns. The less obvious, but equally important, concern is that it should be easy for you to get along with your therapist. You should feel valued and respected, but not judged. The role and responsibility of the therapist will always remain that of a counselor. They will be there to help you find the potential and deep self love within you.

They won't invalidate or minimize your pain. They will only ask for you to understand the source of your pain.

Although there are chances that you may not find the right therapist, don't give up. You will eventually find someone who matches you exactly, and healing won't be far off.

Chapter 3: Ten Somatic Interventions That Can Help You Heal From Your Trauma

"The curious paradox is that when I accept me as I am, I can make way for change."

Carl Rogers

The happily ever after is a common theme in fairy tales. Two fated lovers are bound to find one another through the infinite power of the universe. They fall in love, overcome challenges, and then marry. It's the stuff you only dream of.

Unfortunately, fairy tales rarely account for what happens after the ceremony. It is the years you spend together building your family, raising your kids, and then you realize that the future holds no space for you. It's only you who are enmeshed in their memories. Therefore, you need to make plans that don't involve them. It is heartbreaking. The anger that follows it is valid. It wasn't meant to be this way. It was you and your partner to the end, weathering all the storms together. Your absence from them is the reason for the most severe storms in your life.

When faced with life-altering news, there's a bizarre natural sequence that happens. Some accept it as a part of our lives and refuse to let it go. Others continue their daily lives trying to ignore the pain. Others choose to stop and feel the emotions, to allow them to sink in. Can there be a constructive solution? Yes. Yes.

The importance of body-oriented psychotherapies in post-traumatic stress management is increasing. These therapies are subsets that focus on the brain and body. This makes sense if you think about simple things such as eating chips if you don't feel hungry. Your body doesn't tell you to have the chips. Your body knows when it is full. The mind is what tells your body to feel full and to eat more. Once you are aware of this relationship, you will be able to better understand and heal what influences your body and its reactions.

The best thing about somatic therapy? It can increase self-awareness as well as improve the way you interact with others. You may notice an increase in your awareness of your body and how it responds to pain. This will help you find ways to ground yourself, reduce stress, frustration, and look for signs of emotional turmoil.

Do you think there are any methods that somatic therapies can work? Yes. You can cope with trauma by using a number somatic interventions. We'll now discuss ten of them.

How to Develop Somatic Awareness

Sometimes, the many reasons our bodies activate their distress systems can be so complex that it is difficult to understand or apply common logic. These symptoms can be described as medically unexplained. These are Medically Unexplained Symptoms. In somatic psychotherapy, people are first taught about the science of body awareness and how they may nurture it. Body awareness describes the level of consciousness you possess and the extent to which your mind is connected with your body. It is an awareness of the position and flow of your body, in response to nerve centres, joints and muscles. This is the key to grounding. Because your joints and muscles communicate information about your body with your brain which can then influence how you move. It gives you an understanding of where your body is in space. (Goldstein, 202). It allows you to see objects and people around, their distance and position in relation to you. This helps you understand your stress and pain at the cellular level. Are there thoughts that are too restrictive? Are there objects in your environment that can trigger you? Understanding and answering these questions requires somatic awareness. It can also help you determine which thoughts or behaviours will nourish you and bring you back to the forefront. By understanding the sensations of your body, you can initiate healing and changes that feel physical.

This is a simple exercise that you can do right now: Sit down on a chair with your feet on the floor. Check the alignment of the spine against the chair. Pay attention to the sensation of your bottom. Is your bottom comfortable or does it need to be re-aligned? You can adjust your body until it is completely relaxed. Keep your feet flat on a hard surface. You can look around and observe the surrounding environment. They could be as simple and mundane as a table, to as elegant as a window looking out onto a patch of natural beauty. What are you feeling right now? You can center that feeling for 2 minutes and then go back to what you were doing. While your grief may not return immediately, it will come back at random moments throughout the day.

Re-sourcing

The ability to source is a way of increasing safety and stability. It is a conscious effort by us to invite our minds and bodies into allowing good feelings to flow through, such as the feeling of safety. This will help you to remember that even in difficult times, there are always people and things that will support you. Family, friends, children and loved ones, strengths in art and work (or singing), happy experiences, a basic safety blanket and safe spaces that give you the feeling that no harm will befall you, that there is peace, quiet, and calm. Resourcing allows you to access comfort resources during trauma. This is a great way to have someone to turn to in times of grief. We recall the emotions that we associate with these comfort resources, so that our mind and bodies can heal and recover. This is the water you have to call upon in times of emergency and extreme thirst.

Try this simple exercise: Sit down in a comfortable place and try to think of something that makes your heart happy. It might be a happy moment, like the time you took your children along to a special location and ended up having a lot of great fun. It can act as a blanket that you can touch to feel grounded and comfortable. Take note of what it might be and keep it in mind. Keep this memory in your mind and experience the feelings associated with it when you are feeling overwhelmed by grief. You will feel more secure if you do this.

Grounding in the Present

Grounding can be used to help your body develop its innate senses, ground your feet on the earth and calm your nerve system. It is a powerful trauma management tool that can calm your emotions. Grounding helps us to relax and balance our neuronal networks when we are feeling too stimulated or provoked. You can use tools that help to regulate and calm down our mental and physical health. Grounding is a sense that you are present, and can help you return to the present if your thoughts start to spiral downwards.

Simple grounding exercise: Two bowls are needed. One bowl should contain warm water and the other one should contain cool water. First, dip your hands in the coolwater. Let the cool water flow over your fingers. Take note of the temperature, the amount, and how you feel. After one minute, you can take your hands out from the cold water and place them in a bowl filled with warm water. Keep your focus on the present moment. That is, the act and sensation of touching the water.

Descriptive language is used

Modern somatic therapy encourages you to become more curious about the state of your body and mind while you grieve. Sometimes, the mere pain of recalling these experiences makes it difficult to recognize them. However, to truly heal, one must be aware that these experiences are happening. Traumatic memories or anxiety can be dealt with more effectively if the person is able to connect with, articulate, and allow the feelings to flow through them. There are many adjectives you can use to describe your feelings, such as: hot, numbing, freezing; sharp, throbbing; and dull. Let me explain with an example. Let's assume that you have been hurt in a fall. It causes hot pain and inflammation around the area. After a while, the pain becomes duller and aches. What do you think I am doing? To give you an actual physical dimension, I use words like "hot", and "dull".

It is possible to learn more about how our bodies work by paying attention to what we feel. As we age we become more sensitive and sensitive to the signals that let us know if something might be dangerous or unpleasant. Imagine that you discover a new trekking route. But, when you feel the discomfort, your hair will stand up and give way to goosebumps. It is possible that we have strong feelings of resentment about this course. Our intuition tells us when something is wrong. If we can trust our instincts, our connection with our inner self will grow stronger. Our ability to spot these signs is both instinctual and extraordinary in its reliability. As long as we believe in our senses, we will be able to perform the necessary actions to feel safe and secure.

One thing to do: Try associating a descriptive term with your next sadness. Perhaps sadness makes you numb. Start by feeling that numbness. Is it coming from your chest or elsewhere? Does it cause your body to ache or numbness? You can then say, "A numbness started in my stomach, and then I felt my legs and hands start to hurt." This will help to clarify how you feel in the moment. It can also be used to ground yourself.

Somatic Movement

You can use movement to help your body navigate past traumas, frustrations, and difficult situations. It can help you feel closer to yourself and others and give you confidence that things will turn out well. Somatic movements are performed with total consciousness. The sole purpose of somatic movements is to be aware of how you feel when you perform the movement. It is essential to practice it slowly in order to be the most effective. The human nervous system is responsible for the movement and postures we make. It's possible to improve your movement speed over time with practice. You can also increase the pace at which you perform the movements while maintaining a level of consciousness about what you are doing.

Somatic movements believe that in order to be fully effective, a practitioner should focus more on their internal experience than the outcome. I am reminded of the lyrics to a very popular Beatles song. This line came from an iconic quote in The Readers' Digest 1957 edition. It was written by Allen Saunders. It goes that life is what happens to us when we're busy making plans. We have become so used to looking at the results of what we do that it becomes difficult to actually enjoy the process. The result is that our lives become a collection of definite outcomes. And we forget how much effort and motivation we invested in the journey. Somatic movement asks you to return to your consciousness. To feel the act, you must let it follow its path.

Try this little exercise: Lay down on a floor mat. Your back should be flat. Keep your spine straight. Close your eyes. Your hands should be at your sides. Now relax your muscles. Now breathe in through your chest. Hold this position for a second. Then, exhale out through your stomach. As you do this movement, pay attention to the inner cycle that runs through you. Repeat this ten more times.

Self-Regulation, and co-regulation

The basis of our human experience is connection. If anything is to last, it must be connected. We all desire to be understood, and we all long to be seen. When we build relationships, we want to feel part of the group. When it comes down to overcoming trauma, the autonomic neurological system (ANS), which controls how our environment influences us and how we navigate stress, plays a crucial role.

Somatic regulation is a way to calm ourselves by connecting to the outside environment. It also allows us to use the ANS as a tool to manage our stress levels. This becomes easier if we can relate to an external object's language of love, or the language o warmth and stability. If it's the same language we love, then lifelong connections can be made. However, somatic selfregulation is the method that we use internally to relax and avoid external influences. To survive in real life, both of these regulations are crucial. It is important that we can calm ourselves and be able rely on others for comfort and safety in stressful situations. Self-regulation helps to identify the root cause for destabilizing feelings. Co-regulation relies on close relationships to provide a balance in your healing. The idea of emotional regulation, which helps us respond to spontaneous events without having to lose our inner selves, is at the core of all this. It helps us live with more meaning, to love abundantly, and to find joy even in the smallest things in life.

You can try this: The next time you feel down, pick up the phone to call a friend. Remember a positive memory you shared with them. Tell them your current situation and how they could help. Being open to other people's help is essential if you wish to be seen. Love is always the best solution.

Titration, Pendulation

Every emotion we refer to is associated with a sensation. Consider it. Anger makes us feel hot and clammy. Panic can lead to sweaty eyes. Sadness leads to a prolonged sleep period and dull feelings. All emotions can be expressed using a physical sensation. It can become overwhelming if you feel too many of a particular sensation. Because our survival mechanism (the fight/flight response) is programmed into our minds, our minds will pay more attention to danger than to safety. Because of years of trauma, if we keep adding to our threat systems and fail to address them, it can lead to an emotional breakdown. The possibility of this happening increases if there are years of negative experiences that have accumulated over time.

Somatic therapy is a holistic approach to healing. It requires you to view your body from a body-centered viewpoint so you can give the right outlets to the emotions you are trying to release. These two methods include pendulation or titration.

Titration can be described as the act of slowing down. It requires you to not react quickly and haphazardly to events, but to take your time and develop a slow response. You are in control of how fast you react to events.

By slowing down your response, you take in only a little bit of what you have been given, then you slowly absorb it, so that your activation, arousal, and activation reactions can process this bit. Next, you will respond to another bit. Your body will slowly release tension. Pendulation helps you move between two states. The natural order of the world works in a similar way. We have day and night, ebb-flow, high and low tides, high and lower tides. Pendulation centers your body and puts a little stress along with some

51

relaxation. You can alternate between stress-related and nonstress related.

You should always have someone to assist you with this activity.

Act Of Triumph

An act of triumph can be used to refer to a catastrophic shock or event in which the body fails to protect itself. It then compensates by learning to use the protective mechanism again at a later stage. This is the result a collection of past experiences getting stuck in the system. These previous experiences manifest as invasive visuals, feelings anxiety terror, fear, emotional instability and a sense of sadness or hopelessness. A single case of trauma can be described as the act of victory. It is the accomplishment of an incomplete act that couldn't have been completed at that time.

It could also mean, hypothetically speaking, that one has the desire to support himself with his hands during an unanticipated injury but is unable to do so. While it would be natural to want to flee at the accident site, or because you were caught off guard, it could also mean that your instinctive response is not to do so. Traumatic experiences do not always look at the incident but instead examine the way that individual bodily reactions to the event are mediated.

While you may be out of that particular traumatic situation now, your body's components-your cells-are still tied to it. You feel relief when you are able respond to it. Let's consider a hypothetical situation in which something you should have said no to years ago was not possible. To say "no" would be an act that is a triumph. It would allow you to feel the reality of the situation and know that if it were up to you, your answer would be "no". This can be followed up with a feeling of relief and acceptance.

Consider this: What was the last time you were really mad? It doesn't mean you have to be mad about it. Remember the moment you were angry and what it was. Next, take a pillow and kick it as hard as possible, keeping the memory alive. Say to yourself, "I am capable of handling this."

Sequencing

Have you ever seen dominoes played? There are many tiles that are lined up in a particular order. They all stand close together but they don't lean towards each other. If the player flicks the end a line dominoes, they all fall in rapid succession.

By sequencing, tension can be released and allowed to vent. It begins with one side of your body, and works its way up to the rest. It can feel like you are breathing deeply. This simple movement requires that you only use your stomach or nostrils. However, it can have calming effects on your mind.

It is obvious that all of us experience anxiety. These moments can be pit-sinking and stomach-lurching. As a result, our bodies become clammy and we feel cold. You will begin to feel the tension build up in your throat and constrict your forehead. The anxiety can often ease over time. It will first leave our foreheads, then move to our feet and fingertips, and finally, our whole body. Restricted peace is left behind. Once this happens, we feel lighter in our hearts and can begin to return to our normal states.

One exercise: Next time your anxiety is intense, try sitting quietly in a recliner. Feel the anxiety. It is moving in your body. Is it from where? Is it moving anywhere? Breathe deeply for at least two minutes. Visualize the anxiety leaving your system. You can think of it as the gradual shedding of your work-clothes. Then, you will settle into something more comfortable in the morning. Breathe deeply until you feel calm.

Setting Boundaries

You cannot heal unless you know where your boundaries are. Our daily lives often make it difficult to see when we are doing enough. It is also important to know when it is okay and appropriate to say no. This can lead to long-term problems. This includes ourselves. You may have had days when you worked hard even though you knew it was too much. This is just one instance. However, the point is to be able to recognize when it is okay to not do any more than what you already have.

A little bit of advice: Look in the mirror and say "no". Loudly and clearly say it. As the word rolls in your mouth, imagine a situation when you would have used it. Try to imagine that situation and you might be able to say no the next time.

Now, we are at the end of this chapter. Have you been carefully reading the chapter? Do you still haven't read this carefully? It might take some rereadings for all the concepts to sink in. Slowly read the following words. Allow the words to sink in. Visualize your mind comprehending your abundance and the goodness it brings you. Take a deep, slow breath and slowly reread the information. You can think about how to make the movements part of you mind and body by absorbing them. Yes, your identity has been shaped by grief. However, this does not mean you cannot heal.

Next chapter will focus on somatic exercises. This is where you can release tension from different parts of your body. This is most likely due to the trauma of grief. Once you learn how to release the tension, you'll find peace.

Chapter 4: Somatic Mindfulness Exercises

Trauma can be one your most difficult and challenging things to heal. Trauma can feel as raw and painful as a deep wound in the flesh. The trauma can fester and cause more pain for many days or months. Stress situations can cause emotional and psychological trauma. They are usually triggered by events that question your identity and leave you feeling overwhelmed and helpless in a world with everything out of control. A daily assault of emotions can make it difficult to feel physically painless. This can cause a loss of your connection to others. The trauma will only get worse if it is accompanied by fear and hopelessness.

As an example, trauma can mean that you no longer do the normal things you used to do before the traumatic event. However, you feel confused and lost. Things no longer taste the same. You are no longer able to enjoy things that used give you pleasure. Even getting out from bed can make your head spin and cause weak bones. However, this should not be the case as you know there are no "clinically" problems with you. Trauma can grow in your bloodstream and cause damage to your body.

Each person responds differently to trauma and uses different wavelengths. We need to realize that there is no correct or proper way to react to trauma. Don't compare your way of dealing with trauma with someone else's.

It is important to remember that the situation is personal. The way you respond is your normal response in an abnormal situation. Some of the emotional reactions include guilt, denial and anger. Other symptoms include body pain, breathlessness and muscle spasms. Some people feel all or some of these things. Others may feel only a few. Whatever your feelings, it doesn't matter what they are. It is crucial that you find a way of getting through it so that you have a chance to live normal. The trauma can be caused by any number of things, including a single incident or disruptions to your emotional and physical health. However, it is still the same feeling.

The use of somatic exercises, which are grounded in mindfulness and sensory awareness, can help you cope with trauma. It is important to keep your attention focused on what you are doing. This can help you find some direction and hope in a dark time. Somatic awareness helps to improve your body-mind relationships and your ability monitor your emotions. This can assist in the healing and resolution of traumas that are most severe or debilitating. You can identify whether you were in the flight, flee, and freeze reactions by allowing your body the space and time it needs. If this continues to fester it may cause prolonged psychological stress, as well trauma-related symptoms. In these cases, somatic mindfulness suggests that you pay more attention to mindfulness. Meditation can also increase your connection to your body's core sensitivities.

Individuals in distress are more likely than others to shut down their senses and suppress sensory inputs. The response to trauma or fear cannot be stopped, and the stress and internal fear will continue. Our brain responds to trauma and fear, which has a direct impact on our physiological health. By reacting to stress by suppressing our inner grief, and refusing to let go of it, we allow it to fester within us. This can cause more internal stress. If the nervous systems is not able to regulate our internal emotions and we continue to be in situations of high arousal or irritation, tension can develop. Unreleased grief is still stored in the system and manifests as muscle spasms, depression, and paralyzed states. Somatic mindfulness encourages us to find outlets for this stress and not let it deplete us internally.

We lose the ability to see what our bodies are feeling at any given moment if our nervous system is constantly being internally suppressed or stimulated. This is quite sad when you think about this deeply. We only have one life. This is a gift. Is a gift worthless if it is forgotten and placed in a corner? What good is it to allow dust and other debris to build up on a gift until the day when we are unable even remember how beautiful it was? If you allow mindfulness and somatic attention to enter your body, you bring your presence-your soul back into it. We say that the body can be considered a temple or a place where you can worship your inner divine spirit. Most people take years to find this connection. If you look at it, it is all in the small things. You can find little things that will help to remind you of who you are and how valuable your inner self is.

Understanding mindfulness is about being present and aware in every moment. This may sound simple, but it's one of most rewarding and difficult things you'll ever learn. Humans have a tendency to set unreasonable standards for themselves and to constantly measure up to them. When we fail to meet our standards, or take a small step back, we feel guilty. Instead of jumping into "what if-s", somatic mindfulness asks that you just be, in all your consciousness. Let's start with something simple.

Close your eyes and imagine how you feel right now. Feel the pulse and sensations of your life.

* Next, take in all of your surroundings. They can be anything you want. You can just accept them as they currently are.

* Try to stand straight up, and breathe evenly. Focus your attention on the body. Your heels should not touch the floor.

* Once you have waited for about a minute, get up on your toes and feel the changes in your posture. Return to your feet.

* Keep your rhythm slow, and your breathing steady. Pay attention to the sensation of your hips, lower back and heels touching the ground. Remain relaxed.

Keep going until your heels touch the ground. This will allow you to focus on the fact that you are losing a lot of emotional baggage. While this may sound simple, you need to be patient and take the time to feel your weighing emotions leave your body and run through the ground underneath. Be aware that you're on a journey for self-rediscovery and healing. Every small step is a significant one.

With that in mind, here are some exercises to consider.

Step 1 - Wave Breathing

* Stay still with your mind firmly focused on the moment. Place your hands on the fronts of your thighs.

* Breathe deeply. Notice how your breath flows. Is it rapid or slow?

* Keep your breathing slow and keep your chin up as you inhale.

* Gently glide your hips inwards. Then, lean forward with your upper body. Your eyes should be focused in front of you.

* Now, take a moment to breathe in. Lower your head and inhale.

* Now, slowly move your hips forwards and return to an upright posture.

* Repeat this eight times. Keep your eyes on the steps at all times and keep your mind focused on the flow of your own body.

Step 2 - Bamboo Swaying

Relax and feel at peace. Breathe deeply.

* Gently sway your body backwards or forwards as though you're a tree being pulled along by a gentle breeze.

* You may experience little shudders during the movement. This indicates that your body has released tension. You should take this feeling slow.

* Recover your original position and inhale deeply after two minutes. Pay attention and observe your inner being. Is it any different? Do you feel more relaxed now?

Step 3: Quiet Flow

* Stop and let your vision blur. Defocus.

* Slowly move forward, and your left heel will come to the ground in front.

* Now shift your entire weight into the front right foot. Make sure the right foot is still back exactly where it was when the movement began.

* Open your fingers and reach out to your left arm.

* Once your left heel touches the ground, extend your left arm to make a fist. Breathe in.

* Pause for one minute, then stand up again. Now, relax your left hand and bring it back to its original position. Breathe.

* Perform the movement on the left side of you body twice and then switch. When you are performing the movement, keep your mind and body open to all aspects of your breathing, including your movements and

consciousness. Do not let your movements feel chaotic.

* Do the repetitions until you feel comfortable with your body. Are you more relaxed and conscious of your current state of being? Do you feel alive? If so, where does this sensation come from? Pay attention, as this sensation is necessary to heal.

Step 4 - Breathe of Life

* Stand up straight and concentrate on your breath. Now take a deep inhale. Then, release your breath and make the sound "shh" with your lips.

* Make loud noise. Notice how your stomach feels between your chest and stomach. Continue making a loud noise until you lose your breath. Next, breathe in. Repeat this exercise for 8 more times.

* The sound'shh!' can be used to expand the diaphragm. If it's tight or locked up in conditions of absorbed anxiety, it can hinder

our breathing. By opening it, we can move from a stagnant state to an active one.

* Take a deep, slow breath. Make a gentle "hmm" sound when you exhale, almost as if your sighing is being heard. Keep your lips close together.

* Try to locate a pressure point in your mouth that produces maximum vibrations when you make the sound. You can continue until you run out, then stop and breathe in.

* Repeat for eight times, paying attention the sensation of vibration.

* The vagus neuron, the primary branch of the parasympathetic nerve system, is activated by a humming sound. It helps in the repair and maintenance of overstimulated nervous cells, which allows us to rest.

* Take a moment stand and pay attention to any physical sensations. Allow any trembling, shivering, or the desire to stretch to unfold.

* Can your senses tell you if your breathing has changed? What does this look? Is it possible to put it into words?

Step 5: Taking control

* Our bodies are prone to becoming trapped and losing their natural flow when certain parts of our bodies become too tight or stiff. It is important to be aware of these moods and use techniques that intentionally create and release tension. This practice allows you to pay attention to the actions of your neurons, allowing them to detect stiffness and then help it transform. You must stand still in order to do this movement. Breathe in.

* Tend to the muscles of different areas of your body. You can begin by tightening your neck muscles and throat muscles. Many of us have stress stored in these areas. This is an unconscious accumulation or tension. The movement helps to release it.

* Now, clench your arms. Next, move to your shoulders.

* Third, clench and squeez your stomach. Many people feel tightening in their stomachs because of worry. However, others feel emptiness or an absence. It may be possible to feel more calm and connected to your body by connecting to your gut.

* Now, you need to clench your fists. Many of us feel disconnected from our limbs. This can be a problem because it is our legs that connect us with the earth and help us make instant decisions (e.g., physically removing ourselves from an area of harm). Feeling grounded is all about connecting to your legs.

* Slowly count up to eight breaths, keeping the tension intact.

* Exhale slowly and deeply at the eighth breath.

* Do this again from the beginning.

* A suggestion: As though all cells are glowing, imagine that the body area you are tensioning as you breathe in. For 8 counts, let go of your breath and imagine the area

becoming soft like butter when you heat it. Repeat the process twice for each region. You may find it beneficial to close your eyes when performing this movement. However, that depends entirely on your physical comfort. It's also possible to do it with your eyes wide open.

Step 6 - Swing

* Slowly move your upper back from side to side while you stand still. Your movement should look over your right, then left shoulder.

* Rotate your body as you go.

* Relax your arms. You should follow the movements of your body. Your arms should move gently while you perform the movement.

* Relax your knees and allow your pelvis to twist slightly.

* Move slowly and notice how your spine moves. You should do this for about one

minute. Examine how you feel at the moment. Do you feel calmer, more present, or your energy has changed?

Somatic grounding, resourcing visualization, self control, and body scanning are some other ways to experience somatic awakening (Aybar 2002). Let's go over each one briefly before we end this chapter.

* Grounding. As we have discussed, grounding can help you refocus on your present situation. This is a great method to take your mind off the things that cause your pain. It can help to get back in the present from traumatizing flashbacks or heartache.

Be comfortable with your body and how it feels at that moment. This could be moving to one side or the other, slow running, or stretching your legs and hands. Be aware of your breathing. Control your inhalation as well as your exhalation. Keep inhaling for two seconds until you reach a count of five. Now exhale, for a count five. Each inhalation should be followed by a safe sentence. This should be something that provides comfort, such as "I am safe/I'm there/ It's okay".

* Categories: Have a fun game of "categories". Choose a particular letter, like "b". Next, recall five words belonging to a certain category that begin with the letter b. In other words, you could choose to pick the category food and the five words would be bread, blueberries (butter), banana, bread, bacon, and blueberries. You can take your time and choose the words you want.

* Visualization plus Resource: Resourcing requires you to attune yourself to sensations not related to what you are currently experiencing. This can be quite a difficult process, and you will need to seek the guidance of a professional therapist. But you can begin some exercises at-home that will help you get started. These techniques can help you relieve tension in your body, especially if stress emotions and thoughts are present.

It is possible to begin them by doing so when you are not stressed. It is better to start something when it is not stressful. If you're feeling overwhelmed or stuck, it can be easier to create the same sensations later.

Create a safe space for yourself in your mind. This can be achieved by returning to a location and moment when you felt safe and content. You may even find a new safe refuge that you have never been to before. Be open to the possibilities. Take a moment to feel your limbs. Pay close attention how relaxed you are. You might also consider people who make it easy and make it happy. You could start by looking at photos or focusing on common experiences.

* Self-Regulation. Trauma that is left untreated may cause disturbances to the autonomic nervous. This could indicate that you are always on alert. In this situation, you might react to stress or anxiety as well as other people or situations in ways that may be linked to your traumatic experiences.

Emotional self-regulation refers to the act of managing your emotions to alleviate discomfort. Somatic therapy helps to regulate self-regulation by centering the nervous systems. It may help to work with your body and senses in order to shift stress-inducing tendencies.

Give yourself a hug. This is a safe way to hold your emotions and body in check. This is done by placing your left hand across your chest, while your right hand rests on your chest. Your right arm should be crossed over your left shoulder. Keep your left hand in contact with your right shoulder blade. Now, breathe deeply and say something safe like "I'm in the moment". I am safe."

You could also tap or squeeze different parts. While doing this, hold your hand in an open position. This will help you feel secure and grounded.

* Compassionate Touch of the Body: Finally, active meditation can be done by scanning your body to find different signs. Three deep,

relaxing breathes are enough to calm you down if you become stressed. Retire to a comfortable, closed-eye position.

Keep your eyes on your lower torso. Be aware of the way your feet feel on concrete, as well how your pelvis, pelvis, and knees feel. You can feel the comfort of the gentle weight and touch from your hand by gently pressing your palm against your chest.

To test a variant you can put your hands on the chest with both of your hands and notice the difference between this and the position where one hand touches your chest. The sensation of your hands touching your chest is amazing. If you wish, you could draw little circles while holding your palm to your chest.

Notice how your chest rises or falls with every exhalation. Let this feeling last as long you like.

Now, this is the end of this chapter. This chapter is a lesson in compassion. It helps you to take stock of your body and find your inner, intrinsic self. You can also learn to be compassionate about the pain you have suffered. You can use the exercises to be a gentle mother helping her children take care of themselves. The idea is to not be harsh or admonishing. Instead, look for ways you can become more aware and connected to your inner light and deep inner potential. In the next chapter we will explore different somatic techniques to help you cope with emotional triggers or negative emotions. We will also examine different methods of healing from emotional stress-related chronic pain.

Chapter 5: Somatic Exercises To Process Triggers And Heal Chronic Pain

Hazel said, "Grief doesn't make you change," It reveals your true self."

John Green "Paper Towns"

Grief is not accompanied by an announcement or a plan. It doesn't let you know that it will arrive at your door on the next day, so be ready. Life strikes at full-force, so there's an old saying. It's a sad way to feel, with all its emotions. But it's not all hard days. There are days between when you get up in the morning feeling a bit more ready to tackle the day. The coffee tastes less bitter, and the world is brighter. The next morning, when you go to wash your hair, you inhale the shampoo your lover used. It is one the most horrible things that can happen.

The problem with grief is that it doesn't follow a schedule. For example, you could feel very miserable for a year, but then you'll wake up one day later and realize that you have enough and that you can continue living your life. However, this feeling could be felt after a week. Or a month. Or fifty months. Maybe five years. It doesn't invalidate your rights. Even through the grief and pain, you continue to wake up every day, even though it is so difficult. Even if it seems like you might want to give up, you won't. You are a strong, inborn force that pushes you through every day, stronger than you were before.

You are human, dear reader. This is what your spouse would want for you.

It is crucial to encourage your body's ability to heal and be a source of strength over time. So how can you help? Let's start with the present. I want you to pause everything you are doing now and just focus on your posture. What's the root cause of your tension? Are you at ease or are you causing tension? Are you at ease? Are you slouching in your chair? If you're struggling with anxiety or trauma or are experiencing negative emotions, it can be hard to believe your body is working in you favor. There is no stopping your journey to recovery once you've achieved this.

You should pay attention to small details like your posture, how your breathing is, or if your heart beats too fast.

* Next, search for obvious signs and symptoms of stress. Is it tightness in your gut or discomfort in your shoulders? A migraine? Numbness in fingers?

* Next, consider explicit and implicit factors that contribute positively to your sense of well-being. In one sentence, describe a favourite garment, food or setting (beach, couch, etc.) and a moment with that cherished one.

* Next, consider what external triggers are most likely that you will be triggered. What do people think about noise, shadows, or darkness at night, as well as going out to meet people and attending social events.

Your body should be likened to a favorite book. Something you are familiar with deeply, but also something you can refer back to to improve your understanding. When you start to listen to your inner voice, you will create a permanent channel for communication with your body. This will enable you to find, contact, and overcome trauma situations. This is where you can understand what is happening and how your mind, body and brain are responding to it on a physical and physiological level. This six-step, somatic exercise (Goldstein & 2021b) will help you to get started. This will help you keep track of what could happen in future trauma situations.

* Recognize where you are at the moment. Take a few deep inhalations and exhale. You should pay attention to your feelings inside and out. Note the speed with which you breathe, how your heart beat is, and what temperature your body is at.

* Think of a moment of safety. Imagine a time when you felt the most happy, secure,

peaceful, and fulfilled. Take a moment to remember that time.

* Assess your current health. * Identify the moment and/or location in which your body was affected by stress. You can write it down if you need.

* Now think about how you transitioned from a peaceful state to one of stress. Take a moment to slow down and consider how the event changed from peaceful to stressful. As you replay these events, pay close attention to any statements, objects or attitudes that made you feel anxious, uncomfortable, or both.

* Keep an eye out for things. You should be alert to any changes in your sense of smell and taste. Slow down and pay attention to any changes in your body temperature.

* Healing with your hands. Your palm should be placed on the affected region. Take a deep, slow breath. You can also place your hands on your heart to calm down and allow

yourself to feel that you are still here. You are simply existing.

These stages should be used to assess if your body is changing or shifting. Even if you find things are the same, it is OK. Being more present and grounded can be as simple as tuning in to your inner feelings and sensations.

The philosophy behind somatic therapies is that there are many ways to heal. Your body will do what is best at the moment. Because each person is unique, the healing process that results from learning to accept this philosophy can last a lifetime. This is not only about the healing aspect, but also because this therapy encourages the acceptance of your inner self to unlock your full potential. It does more than just heal you. It also brings out all your glory.

It is common for emotional pain to manifest as pain in the body and joints. We learn to accept the fact that suffering is a part of our lives. This will happen regardless of how we respond. But somatic therapy can help us realize that we have all the tools necessary to make a difference. This is why somatic therapy can help you understand the causes of emotional distress. Understanding the cause of your pain is key to finding relief. An experienced somatic therapist can help identify the cause of your pain and guide you towards finding relief. The only way to resolve your problems is through treatment. You can also read this chapter to prepare you for your first meeting with your therapist.

You may be concerned that therapy might bring about changes that you aren't ready for. Somatic therapy's methods are carefully integrated and introduced slowly and gently so that you can express the pain you feel. April Lyons states in a blog post, Psychotherapy Boulder, that this kind of expression is able to bring back hope that may have been lost (Lyons 2020). Dear reader, you will find that hope is very powerful. Hope gives you strength and confidence to take the next step in your life.

With your therapist, you will be able to work together to address your chronic emotional pain.

It is possible to start by being more aware of yourself. Somatic therapy will teach you how to be more in touch with your body. Somatic therapy teaches you how different parts of your body feel and react to pain. It also reveals how they interconnect. You will be able learn to sense different sensations related to stress, such as how you breathe, how fast your heart beats, how your fingers respond when memory is recalled, and how tired.

Think of your body in terms of a totality of its parts. They are not independent from each other. Let's think about this hypothetically. Beautiful chocolate/candies are a magnet for our senses. We are drawn in by the rich colors and delightful scents. Beautiful bars, nestled between shiny paper covers, are beckoning to our senses. They didn't just come straight out of the bean. Their creation was influenced by many processes. Did you ever try the original seed from a cacao tree? I have, and I recommend that you never make the same mistake. It is bitter.

So the seeds go through a fermentation process to give them a firm flavor. They are then dried and roasted. Once the shells are removed, cacao nibs can be made. These are ground to create pure chocolate. All other ingredients are added at this stage: milk solids (butter), nuts, and so on. The chocolate is created at ideal temperatures to give it the perfect body and fine crack when you bite in it. As with this exquisitely made bar, it takes time, love, effort, and hard work to reach your full potential. We are not referring to someone's potential wasted potential when we say they are "a diamond in a rough". This is not a slur, even though we recognize that times are hard. But, you can reach in and use the time as a welding agent to shine.

Somatic therapy helps you identify and manage patterns that can cause disruptions and pain. When chronic pain becomes a problem, it grows and stays with you. You feel constantly hurt and it makes it impossible to feel good inside. This is reverse psychology. It can make it more difficult for you to feel the pain. This disrupts your internal mechanism and makes it difficult for you manage the tension. Inability to trigger the parasympathetic relaxation reflex is what causes chronic pain. The parasympathetic nervous response is responsible to relax and digest when the body feels calm, relaxed, or resting. It reverses the function of the sympathetic division when there is a stressful situation. The parasympathetic nervous system slows breathing and heart beat while speeding up digestion. Chronic stress can cause parasympathetic nerve system dysfunction. Are you a milk-maker? One day, it will boil and simmer, then explode. You may experience an emotional breakdown if your body is unable to bear the strain of tension. You can relax your parasympathetic nervous and brain by using meditation, focusing on your breathing and flexing your muscles.

Complete relaxation can indicate a return of greater physiological control, optimum functioning and clarity. This may help you to regain your sense security.

Somatic therapy helps you recognize how your therapist is helping you to see that changes in your expressions such as your posture, facial mannerisms or muscular tension are the result of chronic pain or routine suffering. This will help you connect with your body to calm and soothe your nervous system which is already frayed and overworked. It will also stop you from causing even more pain. By continuing to do this, you will learn to recognize the effects of letting painful emotions fester in your body. This will enable you to take steps to end such destructive behaviors. Not only will you learn to accept and tolerate pain, but also to recognize that it is normal, something that must be expressed and understood in order to ease it. Your body will heal naturally if you see pain that way.

Your therapist can help you find and address the root of your emotional pain or stress, and help bring it to light. You and your therapist will work together to restore your health by confronting any physical fears or aversions that may be restricting your daily life. You may not even know the source of all the pain. Many times we keep the hurt inside until it becomes too much. Your therapist can help identify whether this is the case and explain how you can find the source of your pain. You and your therapist can work together to reduce pain symptoms and improve your control by using sensory inquiry and breathing techniques. This will lead to the progressive release and healing of unprocessed survival energy which can keep you suffering in an endless loop.

One thing is essential in all of this. Believe that your pain will find a solution, that it will get addressed, and that you will have a platform to express yourself. Although it is an easy task, it can be difficult. You need to be conscious about your diet, sleep, and overall health. Your therapist will give you the support and guidance that you need, in addition to this book. This will allow your outer self expression to come out of your inner self. Believe in them. But, more importantly, believe in you.

Here are some simple exercises that can help increase your sense of somatic awareness. These movement patterns highlight the parts of your body that are most susceptible to sensory-motor loss (also called amnesia). As this is the most direct and effective way to control them, focus on developing a full awareness of the movements in these body areas.

You should remember that somatic exercises are primarily about focusing on your internal sensations. Somatic movement awareness is based on the understanding that it targets your nerve system, which in turn calms and improves functionality of your muscles. This means that you don't target your muscles in these exercises. By stabilizing your nerves you are enhancing your muscular coordination. This is the key to maximizing the benefit of somatic movements. If you are not focusing your attention on this you will not get the most out of them. To maximize your benefits, these are some tips.

* Focus your attention on the intrinsic vibrations and feelings of every movement you perform. Somatic movements may help you to identify the areas most affected by sensory motor neuropathy. Sensory Motor Amynesia (SMA), where the nervous response is adaptive and not obvious, cannot be treated using standard medical or surgical interventions. Motor control is lost when motor receptors of our voluntary cortex have lost their orientation or competence to regulate all of the muscles. This may be due to excessive stress and exertion. Somatic movement is a way to restore your inner self, and allow you to operate normally again.

* Make sure to be comfortable when doing somatic exercise. These exercises may be performed on a yoga or other soft surface, so your spine is not stressed. A mattress or carpet can provide both relaxation and protection, which will allow you to unwind. This allows for greater precision in execution as well as perception. The somatic movements can be performed in comfort by those with chronic impairments of agility or endurance. It is best to choose a firm mattress as the more efficient your movements are. Your clothes should feel soft and comfortable. Activewear is unnecessary since you are not training for a marathon. Your clothes should allow you to breathe freely, and you shouldn't feel restricted. The environment should be comfortable and distracting so that you can do the exercises without discomfort.

* Be patient and don't rush. Injury while exercising is unnecessary, dangerous, ineffective, and completely uninteresting. It is important not to push your muscles. This

gives you an opportunity to think about the actions you are making and not just execute them at the moment. If you put in a lot of effort or exertion during aerobic and cardio activities, your brain gets overwhelmed with sensory input that has no relevance to your task of learning to regulate your body. Your learning progresses in an even and steady manner. It will take diligence.

* Being dedicated and motivated is key to improving your movement patterns. For somatic motions however, this is not the case. You must feel every movement. Feel the movement you are creating with your body. Be a part them. Slow down so your brain and neuronal system can take the time to detect what is happening and then respond appropriately.

* Body-pain can occur when the lower back muscles of the sufferer begin to stretch. This is normal, and it will pass after the muscles have had time strengthen. When you feel discomfort, don't push your muscles.

* Seek long-lasting improvements in your comfort, mobility alignment, and overall functioning, rather than temporary fixes for your physical attributes. It is important to be positive in your expectations and to envision the transformation your somatic nervous system can achieve in your daily life.

Somatic Awareness through a Washcloth

This workout will work your core, abdominals, and pelvis. Your core should feel like you are squeezing a washcloth. You can do this sequence while you are closed your eyes to increase the awareness of your body (Binnendyk (2018)

For this exercise, lie on your back in a fetal posture on a smooth surface. You will do the following while in fetal position. Keep your knees bent and your feet at the level of your feet.

* Spread your arms straight and press your right palm down on your left palm.

* Roll your arms in opposite directions using your arms. Your right palm should be up, and your left one should be lower.

* Keep your arms extended each time.

* You could make this a full-body motion by adding the legs.

* Place your hands on the palms of your palms and lower your knees. Then, tilt your head to the palm-up end.

* Reverse the process. Keep rolling your body forward and back in a continuous movement.

* Keep your hands relaxed and notice how your coordination changes when you complete the exercise five to ten more times.

1.1 1.2

1.3 1.4

Somatic Awareness through Dancing (Fig. 2.1-2.2, 3.2.3, 2.5, 2.4)

This fluid exercise only targets the lower body. It focuses on how motion affects the back and limbs.

* Place your legs straight out in front you and lay flat on the floor.

* Take deep, slow breaths and stretch your right leg outwards. Allow your lower back curve slightly.

* Bend your back while twisting, allowing your leg to flatten.

* The cycle should be repeated five more times on each side. Be aware of how mobility affects lower back.

* Pay close attention to where your backbone wants it to be hunched and straightened.

2.1 2.2

2.3 2.4

Somatic Awareness with Skiing (Fig.3.1–3.2,3.3,3.4)

This flowing twisting exercise helps you balance your stomach and back.

* Bend your knees to bend at the knees while simultaneously turning your feet to the left and to the right. To stabilize, do the twist pivoting on both your heels and landing onto your feet.

* Allow your spine to naturally expand and flatten.

* Repeat the dynamic movement on each side five to ten more times, moving slowly and fluidly.

* Be aware of the effects this has on your sides.

* Continue to extend your legs and do the same movement on each side.

* Your back movements should be the same but slightly smaller.

3.1 3.2 3.3 3.4

Somatic Awareness through Arching & Curling (Fig.4.1,4.2,4.3,4.4, 4.5.4,5.4.6, 4.7.4.8)

This exercise will help to open up your spine. Keep your posture relaxed and calm throughout.

* Spread your legs flat on a firm surface.

* Place your left hand on your left side and bring your left knee towards your chest.

* Hold your right hand with one hand, and then place the other behind your head.

* Exhale and raise your head toward the left knee.

* Relax your body. Breathe and straighten your spine.

* Perform this act thrice. Then switch sides.

4.1 4.2

4.3 4.4

4.5 4.6

4.7 4.8

My belief is that you will find success if your goal is to do somatic healing. Every new endeavor is hard. It takes time to get used to the idea of healing and to adjust to it. Although we want to get over the loss of our spouse, there is more. We are also looking for our inner self, our strength, love, and to get back our love of life.

"Life's for the Living" is a song by The Passengers. One section of the song is "Smile For the Living/ Get What You Need and Give What You're Given/ Life's For the Living so Live It ..." Grief makes us forget. We believe that suffering and pain are the purpose of life, and so we forget the good times, the happy moments, and everything else that makes us human. Unintentionally seeking out ways to keep unhappy and in suffering, we become a shell of ourselves. Our goal is find a way to get back to ourselves, to the part of us that is internal and what makes us human. Once we find a path back, once it becomes clear that not being in pain means that we don't have to live a life that isn't worth it, we will be able to see that life is amazing and should be enjoyed.

Next, we'll discuss the emotional rollercoaster associated with grief. This can be one of your most difficult experiences. We'll also be discussing the stigmas and social issues that come with being widowed and how to adjust to your new life. Keep in mind that your life is yours and that you are not responsible for anyone else's decisions.

Chapter 6: Understanding Trauma

W

What is trauma? I keep running into people who know what trauma is, but are often wrongly describing it. Only a fraction of the truth is true. Trauma must be catastrophic, violent, rape-inducing, or similar occurrences. Although such events can be very traumatizing, there are many other things that could be equally as traumatizing. This chapter describes trauma in all its many aspects.

What is Trauma and How Does It Work?

A trauma is a severe mental injury that results in brain damage from extremely stressful situations. These emotional reactions can cause stress reactions that lead to victims becoming overwhelmed and losing control. It often takes some time to process memories and other experiences. Trauma can develop if the experience proves too terrifying or overwhelming. It is possible to evoke the same experience in different situations. This could happen if someone has ever been in an elevator and suffered trauma. They may experience anxiety or panic attacks just thinking about an elevator. Trauma can trigger both strong emotional reactions and physical reactions.

The Greek word "trauma" is where the term comes from. It refers to injury or wounds. The general distinction between psychotrauma (psychological, emotional, or mentally trauma) is made. All terms can be distinguished.

The term trauma in medical practice: Doctors refer to a trauma as a physical injury. A serious injury must preceded by violence or an accident. This form of injury has been documented since 19th century.

Psychotrauma in psychology is severe mental shock. These are situations or accidents (e.g. Craniocerebral injuries can lead to severe after-effects. Traumatizing experiences, like sexual violence, can have devastating effects on body and soul. This describes both the triggering and subsequent complaints. Mental traumatizations have the potential to cause mental disorders. They can also cause excessive stress in the body which can lead to emotional numbness.

The term "traumatizing experiences" is used. This includes wars and rapes, torture, as well as direct attacks on oneself. You feel a combination of helplessness and horror. You may also experience mixed mental and physical trauma.

Some anxiety and stress may disappear by themselves. The ability to overcome trauma is a key factor in allowing people to grow. People affected by trauma are more open to small details of daily life. People may see their lives in a different light after experiencing a physical or psychological trauma. You live more conscious.

Trauma refers to events that have overpowered us and left us feeling helpless. Today, this definition is outdated because not all traumatizing events are characterised as helplessness.

My body may feel traumatized after I have an operation. Suddenly, I experience post-traumatic Stress Disorder (PTSD), which I cannot explain as I don't link it to the event. the operation) at any time.

It is common for sexual violence to be perceived as traumatic when it comes to children. The perpetrator may sneak in. The perpetrator can be very kind and strokes children. But the actions have a devastating effect.

This means that we can't always predict which events might be traumatic because not all events have the same consequences. It's dependent on the state we are in, how the event has impacted our bodies, and not necessarily our minds.

Different types of Trauma

There are several ways trauma can occur. Some can be caused directly by major events, others due to the individual's environment. Stress disorders or traumatic disorders can quickly form, especially when they occur during the child's personality growth.

I will be introducing you to the different types and causes of trauma in the following. Understanding the variety of trauma causes will help us get closer to the answers to the question about what trauma actually is.

People tend to think of shock trauma when they think about trauma. An example of this is when a person experiences an emotion that is overwhelming and leaves them feeling helpless. The person is unable to cope with the trauma. Examples include a divorce, a sudden breakup, or a car accident. The exact cause of symptoms is not always clear.

Developmental trauma, a relatively recent term, is another. It is often based upon older traumatizations that had different effects on the brain and body. It's almost impossible to escape stress situations as a child. This can lead to posttraumatic stress disorder. Stress does not always have to refer to physical violence, sexual assault, or the like.

Trauma can be caused many different situations. Children can become psychologically traumatized when their needs aren't met. You may remember crying for hours as a child when your mother said children shouldn't be spoiled. It can lead to mental disorders, physical ailments and traumatic memories.

Secondary trauma is possible if you work in an emergency room or have been a witness to a traumatic event, such as violence or an accident. These include emergency physicians, therapists, or police officers.

Germany has a phenomenon known as intergenerational trauma, which is caused by the world wars. Many people who experienced wars weren't able to cope with it. This is partly due to a lack of empathy among the postwar generation. Because children were not able to feel comfort after a fall, they were often ignored.

Social trauma refers specifically to events that have a large impact on many people. These include terrorist attacks or train accidents, as well as wars and other such events.

It is possible to have extremely traumatizing effects on our connections if we lose contact with someone. Even small, daily traumas can cause psychological trauma. These include comments that are snide, bullying, and neglect.

Shock Trauma

Shock trauma is the most common definition of trauma. This is a one-time, intense, overwhelming, and unresolvable situation that leaves you powerless and unable to cope with.

It can be, for instance, a car wreck (it doesn't really matter how serious), falls of any sort, visits at the dentist, sudden splits, and divorces. This could include an abortion. These and other similar events may lead to shock trauma. Unfortunately, we don't know enough. Many people experience symptoms but don't know where they are coming. It becomes more complex when we consider developmental trauma.

Developmental Trauma

A developmental trauma is a trauma that has been present for a longer duration, such as if the trauma occurred over several years. But, developmental trauma can occur when the victims are not given enough attention or children are allowed too long to cry and go without being cared for.

It is not clear what the term developmental trauma means. In recent years, shock trauma has been the predominant focus of professional medicine. However, not all symptoms are due to shock. The professional world is more likely to recognize deeper and more long-term traumatizations that can have a profound impact on the body, and the psyche. These symptoms last for longer periods of time due to the fact that we are less likely to be able escape from stressful situations in our childhoods than we are in our adulthood. You don't have need to experience trauma in order to feel symptoms.

One possibility is that our mother couldn't adapt to us, was too scared for us, didn't know how to help us, or let us cry for hours. She believed that children shouldn't be fed or coddled too much. Depressive or narcissistic mothers may also cause developmental trauma in their children.

We will look more closely at the potential effects of traumatization later.

Secondary Trauma

Secondary traumatization is when someone is not directly affected but watches the events as an observer. This could include emergency medical personnel who arrive first following a tragic accident, as well as random witnesses.

Secondary trauma must also be considered when discussing trauma. This applies to people who aid others in emergency situations, or who witness traumatic events.

Emergency physicians, paramedics. Police officers. Firefighters. Therapists. But also, accidental witnesses to violence.

Social Trauma

Social trauma is when many people are affected at one time. This can be the case in natural disasters, terrorist attacks, and other situations. A group of people is affected by the same event. This can result in severe psychological or physical consequences.

Also, sudden severed connections can often be very distressing. It's extremely difficult to say goodbye when we suddenly lose someone.

Transgenerational Trauma

This type of trauma is well-known in the war child generation. When the trauma or fear of the parents is passed to the children, this is known as "war child trauma". For example, parents who have experienced food shortages for a prolonged period of time may urge their children to ensure that they don't cause undernutrition or excess.

Stages of Trauma

The trauma processing phase is usually divided into three phases. These are not all the same for everyone but can be seen in most affected. Traumatization cannot simply be described. It is unique to each individual.

Phase of shock

The shock phase happens immediately after the experience. It can last from an hour up to a week. The amount of psychological support sought and the resilience of the person affected will determine how long it lasts. In order to speed up the process, psychological first aid must be provided. Talk to a friend or relative about the incident.

Phase of Exposure

The exposure phase can last up to two weeks. In this phase, the intense excitement slows down and the events remain vividly in the mind. So-called flashbacks happen when people affected suddenly are thrown back in the memory. Many people affected by this event are completely overwhelmed. This can lead to depression, self-doubt, and feelings of helplessness.

Recovery Period

The recovery phase generally begins after four weeks or 14 days after the trauma. Recovery may be delayed or prevented if there is any other stressors, such a negative attitude of others toward your behavior. If someone is in the recovery stage, they are able to avoid reliving the trauma and can instead look towards the future. People who are affected by trauma often see this as an opportunity to look back and consider the future. For example, victims of terrorist attacks may feel gratitude that they were able to survive.

What if there is no Recovery Period?

If the recovery phase ceases completely, then all living conditions become more stressful. Recurrent memories of the event can appear as flashbacks, nightmares, or flashbacks. As a result, trauma victims avoid anything that might trigger the trauma and have difficulty finding inner peace. The affected should seek professional help if the recovery phase is not completed within the four-week time frame.

Trauma Symptoms

Each person reacts differently to trauma. Some people have only psychological disorders and others are also affected by trauma. Different age groups have different trauma symptoms. Children most commonly suffer from personality disorder and adults are more likely to develop post-traumatic stress disorders (PTSD).

Trauma can also be caused by torture, bad accidents, and separation from your partner. People often try to suppress extreme events like these. This causes an internal anguish. As seen from the outside, traumatized individuals behave very normal, especially at the start. Terrorized people are active and go about their jobs. This however is a fallacy. Because the soul is soon going to get some air. Gloomy thoughts, images and feelings accompany the shock patients through the day and into their dreams. You find yourself drenched in sweat upon waking up and are then confronted with flashes at any time during the day. These are just some of the many trauma symptoms that can occur.

In the mind's Eye, trauma looks like a short film. Emotional and mental disorders such as palpitations or dizziness can be present immediately or weeks later. These symptoms may appear as waves. A person traumatized is often plagued by negative memories. The shock continues to build up for affected people. A tremendous pressure wave builds. Fear and terror are created by harmful stimuli like smells and images. They cause complete passiveness and can't be treated. This causes psychological and physical problems. A vicious circle begins. Let's take a look at the trauma symptoms.

Common Symptoms of Trauma

Trauma symptoms can be described as complaints that result from trauma. This growing suffering can occur in both a psychological and physical way, may last for weeks, years, or even months. Common signs of trauma include:

* Depression

* Helplessness

* Sleep disorders

* Fear

* Hyperexcitability is a constant over-arousal.

* Nightmares

* Jumpiness

* Aggressiveness

* Feeling of isolation

* Stomach, bowel and other problems

* Muscle tension

* Grief

* Rapid breathing

* Fainting

* Cardiovascular disorders

* Dizziness

* Increased sweating

* A lack of concentration

* Loss or interest

* Tachycardia

* General weakness

* Memory gaps

* Flashbacks are memories that come back to you.

* Obsessive compulsive disorder etc.

It can be hard for laypeople to play the role the traumatized person. People in shock often feel misunderstood. They are often considered weak. But, if you take a closer look, you will see that their strength is sufficient to bear the heavy trauma patient burden. Even with good health shock patients have to go through a difficult phase. The effects of trauma on the brain are not similar to those resulting in a cold or a headache.

If the patient is willing to openly share their traumas and work with the therapist on them, the only way to get the memories under control is by revealing the pieces piece by piece. After this bridge of trusting and opening up is reached, you can start to treat the psychological as well as physical symptoms. It may take several sessions before the patient can see clearly again and feels better. There are many factors that affect the length of therapy. It is essential that the emotionally damaged person cooperate with the therapist and have the necessary knowledge.

Symptoms Of Underarousal

The lower end of the amplitude shows certain symptoms we may experience that are part of our daily lives. This is often depression. It is common for depression to be misdiagnosed. They are more likely to be the result of trauma than true depression. Other symptoms include weakness, exhaustion, and listlessness. Escape to other worlds. Food is always helpful, no matter where you are located upstairs or down.

Common is to consume alcohol or to smoke. This can cause you to feel emotional numb and cut off from others.

Symptoms Of Overarousal

On the other end, we find the opposite. We are always in a state of sympathy, i.e. Highest tension. This is often a cause of insomnia.

Many people report feeling exhausted, falling asleep and laying down on the couch. Then, they wake up and find themselves wide awake again.

This is a sign that your sympathetic nervous system isn't able to relax. People often drink beer or wine to unwind. It is also helpful to eat and smoke.

There can be a feeling that you are in a state of inner restlessness. When I ask people if they would just like to sit on the sofa and do nothing, most look at my questioning eyes. You mean, just sitting on the couch and doing absolutely nothing? This is not an option for them. When they calm down, they feel the inner tension and are able to occupy themselves so they don't feel restless.

This condition is often associated with difficulty concentrating. Some people experience panic attacks, anxiety, and panic attacks. Many have difficulty relaxing.

Sometimes they throw tantrums if they get too excited. They can get very upset because everything is a part of their own story. The potential for arousal is always present. People have a tendency to look outside and project reasons for their conditions. They blame the people around them for their conditions.

Hyperactivity can be seen in children as well as adults. Sex addiction can result from its temporary calming effects. Jumpiness, the tendency to move from one idea into another without settling down. You feel like you don't have any direction. These symptoms include a tendency to jump and drama.

Trauma Symptoms for Adults

The traumatized often seeks to return to their normal lives as soon as possible. In rare cases, though, this desire is usually not realized. Because of this horrible experience, the brain will never recover from it. The effects of this massive burden mean that those who suffer from it experience more symptoms. People want to forget this traumatic experience and instead blame the physical causes. They choose to avoid the difficult situation and remain silent. Her memories are still a part of her life. In the end, people affected feel an intense fear that is felt everywhere and every time.

Traumatization can lead to mental disorders such post-traumatic stress disorder. Concomitant problems may include anxiety, eating disorders, or somatoform conditions. Some sufferers try to manage their symptoms using alcohol, drugs or pills.

Four main signs of PTSD are present in adults.

1. The constant sensation of shock, in the form images, sounds and physical sensations, is something that you experience constantly. The stress levels can often be so severe that it causes people to lose touch with reality.

2. Avoid certain situations. People suffering from stress disorder need to avoid places, people, thoughts, emotions, and other situations that may remind them of what happened. Complete withdrawal is possible if fear and depression both increase.

3. Feelings are often lacking during trauma therapy. It's as though their feelings were

destroyed by the violence. They appear completely cut off from the rest.

4. Hyperarousal: An increased sense of urgency and jumpiness. Traumatized people tend to be hyperactive and irritable. They also have trouble concentrating. Traumatization can also cause sleep disorders.

Trauma Symptoms among Children

Particularly difficult for traumatized children is the process of reintegration. Children, unlike adults, are unable understand and process what they've experienced. A traumatized kid may grow up to be an unhappy adult, who struggles to understand the world and has difficulty getting along with other people. The brain of the child is still young. It handles a difficult situation far better than older adults. Post-traumatic Stress Disorder can be caused by traumas or the death in a loved one. Even in children, it is possible to cause serious long-term or short-term harm.

These are the four hallmarks of children with a Stress Disorder:

1. Recurrent memories.

2. You can playfully recreate the traumatic moment.

3. Fears arise as soon as you are reminded of the shock situation.

4. Negative attitudes towards life, mistrust of others and depression.

Some children can be aggressive or hyperactive. Others may wet themselves or bully their family. Each child approaches the experience in a different way. It can be treated in a child-friendly manner that is fun and playful. The best course of treatment depends on the child's symptoms.

What to do if Trauma Symptoms are present

Traumatic experiences can be extremely stressful. It can be difficult to anticipate the effects of traumatization. The better your chances of healing or processing traumatization, the earlier you begin therapy. Being aware of your own trauma should be your first step in coping. Talking with someone trustworthy about the trauma can help you to cope. What caused this emergency? Personal analysis is a great way to minimize flashbacks. You can do it together. Even if the event is not something you feel you can handle, a physician can assess the extent of your trauma and recommend treatment. You can also reprogram the brain by looking ahead and being kind.

Get professional help for Trauma symptoms

Sometimes, the pain is so severe that you cannot manage it on your own. You should seek professional help if panic attacks or depression become too severe. PTSD, or Post Traumatic Stress disorder, should be treated seriously. It is essential that you take steps and let others help you. This is especially important in fighting the burden.

Get Out of the Vicious Circle

The individual responsible must be able to identify the source and deal with the pain as quickly as possible. It is important to actively participate in this process, as it rarely happens by itself. Trauma patients also require a strong and compassionate contact person. This person could be a parent, a friend, or even an expert. It is not unusual to have post-traumatic Stress Disorder. You should seek treatment with a psychiatrist and/or a psychotherapist immediately. Talks with the specialist should soften trauma that may have caused the disorder. Once the patient has spoken to the therapist and doctor, the next step is the processing phase.

The goal of the workup is to extract the repressed hurt so it can be later lit from all sides. This procedure is similar in nature to wound healing. The soul wound also heals internally. However, it is important that the healing process begins before the plaster can go on the wound.

Mental disorders are difficult and require patience, mindfulness and forbearance. It is possible to take small steps backwards during any type of psychological trauma therapy. However, this should not make the individual feel disoriented or helpless. PTSD is easily treatable, especially if the condition is identified early.

What Do You Perceive As Traumatic?

Healthy Nervous System Sympathetic/Parsympathetic Amplitude

Let's first look at trauma: our autonomic nerve system. It includes a parasympathetic as well as a sympathetic branch. They are vibrating at an antagonistic frequency to each other, much like a swing. The oscillation can occur to one or both sides. It is the preferable side that awakens us. This branch is responsible to alertness and arousal. Parasympathetic is responsible in any way for calming.

The Tolerance Window

The tolerance window is where parasympathetic, sympathetic, and parasympathetic branches oscillate. This is the limit between which the amplitudes of the nervous systems oscillate in relatively constant waves between the lower and upper limits.

The distance between them indicates how much we have to work with, how stressed-resistant we are, and how much joy, happiness and excitement we can handle.

The farther these boundaries are from each other and the larger this amplitude is, the stronger we are against stress. Most importantly, we feel happier. The relationships and care of parents or caregivers play a major role in the development of the tolerance threshold (window of tolerability).

Our psychological state is also determined largely by the autonomic nervous. People with a small tolerance limit react quickly to stress or overwhelm situations that are not typical. Some may not be able to fall in love due to the body's inability to regulate stress levels and its reaction with symptoms.

The tolerance window size can be already reduced at birth. People who have had a hard birth, are unwelcome or were pregnant by mothers who were extremely stressed have a highly sensitive stress system. This is more prevalent in those who have experienced a stressful birth than those who had a calm and natural birth.

It has been possible to observe babies for many years and measure their stress levels. Imagine the impact on the amplitude of stress that parents have if they aren't compassionate or unable to understand their child.

What Happens to the Brain in Traumatic Experiences?

Normal memory is where you store the normal events. This allows you to organize it your way in terms both of time and experience. It can be said that emotions and thoughts can still be activated (there and then this and another happened to me... I thought the following and felt it).

A trauma experience can cause a disruption in normal stress processing (safety switches on), and the memory of the trauma is broken up and stored in several areas of your brain. You can quickly relive fragments of your memory by nudging them. Sometimes, traumatized individuals will relive their bad memories in a flashback (as if they were happening again now), like going back to a horror movie at night.

Stress hormones like stress hormones (e.g. Memory functions like learning, memory and storing knowledge. This was true in earlier stages of human evolution (physical reactions such a fleeing or fighting were at the forefront initially, e.g. Fighting for food and fleeing from bears.

Fast reflexes are required for flight and fight. Cerebral interference may have slightly slowed down these reflexes. This may be analogous to a computer that runs more slowly when multiple programs are running simultaneously. The cerebrum proved to be an advantage in survival under certain conditions.

Today's world is not a good place to be. To make decisions in the modern world, one needs to consider complex processes that require the cerebrum to function optimally.

Studies have shown that pregnant women who have experienced extreme stress in pregnancy (flights, violence, fear etc.) tend to be more stressed than their babies. Through the umbilical line, mothers transmit more stress hormones than normal to their babies. These hormones stimulate the development of the stresshormone center. This can then produce more stress hormones for the child over time, perhaps even for their entire lives. The affected person is likely to be more stressed than other people in his life. For example, he may react more aggressively, or feel more afraid, than others.

What Happens in the Body when there is Danger

This is the fundamental requirement that our nervous system functions, and is something we are born with. The moment we find ourselves at the mercy a shocking threat (as defined in shock trauma), our tolerance levels are surpassed. Danger is considered subjective. Sometimes our mind may not be able to recognize danger. However, our body responds to it and the amplitude goes beyond the window. This will be discussed in more detail shortly.

Physical reactions to traumatizing events

Excited, or an acute stress reaction to adrenaline and cortisol being released in the body, heartbeat, blood pressure and heartbeat increase. In addition, small blood vessels under skin close to ensure that injuries don't cause extensive bleeding. The liver releases the sugar reserves so that the body can have more energy. The liver inhibits insulin at this time so that sugar is not immediately destroyed again. The tone is greater in the large muscles while the skeletal muscle tends to be more important. Tunnel vision results when our pupils dilate. Because they are not required at the moment, blood supplies to internal organs, such as stomach and intestinal intestines, are very low. This could explain why so many people who are extremely stressed have gastrointestinal issues.

The Fight and Flight Reflex

This is how our body prepares for fighting or fleeing. Depending on what you do, your body provides the energy.

For instance, if I am walking through a forest and hear a crackling sound in the wood, then my body will first react by orienting itself towards that sound. I discover the reason. Only then can it be decided what I should do. I do not make this decision based on my personality. It is a decision that I make based on the older parts of me brain. Most likely, the decision will favor an escape as fighting with the bear would be futile.

The Torpor

My body is likely to collapse if the bear comes after me. It's futile trying to fight back. The body is in a state of complete shutdown. It is when all energy stops flowing to the body. I then freeze. There are two types: Torpor and trauma.

If I freeze in excitement, I have a lot more energy, but my body is unable to move. The nervous system holds the energy. This is hypertonic.

If the overwhelm lasts a while, I go limp. I then become hypotonic. I stop when I'm completely paralysed. I enter a state known as dissociation. Recently, the term "fawn instinct" has also been mentioned. This is a state where people can stay, meaning that they are happy to make others happy.

A wise man once said that dissociation is nature's grace. While we may be dissociating right now, it is actually us that are actually breaking apart from ourselves. This is impossible to explain.

Many describe it as a near-death experience. They watch each other and aren't connected to themselves. They don't feel the pain or shift in time. You feel like you're a spectator in your own life. A dissociative experience is the most likely sign that symptoms will develop after the situation. Our nervous system is totally out of tune.

Amplitude of a Traumatized Nervous Sytem

Here is an example of how a nervous systems works after trauma. We can see the input vibration. However, it is still within the limits of the tolerance window. The trauma event can be compared to a house equipped with a 220-volt electrical panel that is hit by a 10,000-volt lightning strike.

The whole house becomes flooded with electricity. The human nervous response is the same. We can only manage a certain level in excitement, shock, and fear before our internal fuse blows. At that point, we freeze, stop acting, and surrender.

The problem is the nervous system does not seem to receive any signal to let it know that the situation has ended. The result is that people remain stuck in their current situation. This is because the mind knows it, but the body doesn't know. This is how people are often in an excessively excited state. They are at the highest end of the tolerance range or exceed it.

When people are tired, their nervous systems goes into a state of hypotonic underexcitation and fatigue.

Trauma Management

Trauma therapy usually requires professional assistance. For example, trauma therapy may use the EMDR (Eye Movement Desensitization & Reprocessing), which triggers bilateral stimulation in the brain by using hand movements. The treatment of trauma in psychotherapy is done in several phases.

1. Stabilization Phase: The stabilization stage is where the person involved tries to classify his feelings, and slowly regulate them. It also involves understanding what you have experienced and closing the gaps in your memories.

2. Confrontation phase. This is the second phase. The affected people are confronted by the traumatic event to help them feel better and create closure.

3. Integration phase. During this phase, the affected can be supported to get back to their everyday lives. The therapist evaluates how the person is handling grief and how he is learning how to deal with it.

This is how to cope with trauma

The bad memories you associate with trauma don't have the right to be buried forever. Here are some tips to help you deal with trauma.

1. Talk about it

Talk to someone who you trust about your feelings. You don't have to suppress the experience. Instead, talk about it. Perhaps there are others who have been through similar experiences and can offer support. So you won't feel isolated with your negative feelings.

2. Imagine your achievements

What you've been through so far is what makes you who it is. Traumatized individuals often feel that their failures were their fault, so it is important for them to remember the successes. You can take a piece if paper and list your ten greatest achievements. This will demonstrate that you have achieved much and that you don't need to let trauma ruin your life. By practicing mindfulness, you can learn to appreciate your achievements and believe in positive things.

3. Make friends with people

People affected by trauma often find themselves in isolation after a difficult experience. Don't allow the trauma to drive you insane. Family and friends are important for helping you overcome trauma. You will find that distraction and encouragement are helpful, even though it may seem difficult at the beginning.

4. Find a hobby

If you think you might have an inner artist, a new hobby may be the perfect way to distract yourself from the past. Find something you enjoy and try out other hobbies. If you aren't ready to talk about your trauma yet, painting may help you get through it.

Get rid of your Trauma with TRE

TRE is another technique to relieve inner tension. David Berceli has created a series that combines several exercises which can trigger the neurogenic-tremor. Cordula Paar describes in an interview how this healing process works and how she has experienced a profound change in her life.

Resistance and Resources

The basic condition of a person determines the effect of an event. The tolerance window size indicates how resilient a person is. Mental resilience, also known as resilience, is a measure of psychological resilience. It is the ability to endure and manage situations without giving in.

The term comes originally from materials research. It refers to how much material can be bent, and then returned back to its original state.

Resistance is determined by the resources that we have. All of these are what give us strength, stability, and support: Money, Education. Work. Skills. Talents. Friends. Community.

The two greatest resources, apart from romantic relationships, are relationships and a network of social contacts. And, on the flip side, is the belief in the value of the world, or life.

It is easier to categorize and give meaning to the terrible events that happen in our lives. It is much harder for us to bear when we live in a random universe where everything has meaningless.

The Rollercoaster of Trauma Effects

Many sufferers feel like they are on an emotional roller coaster, as their nervous system oscillates between under-excited and over-excited. You feel trapped and you can't break out of this state of exhaustion or tension.

Once we reach arousal, the window is closed for tolerance, we can be in the realms or flight and fighting. This tension is not good for our social life as we can become much more anxious. By moving within the window, we become more in touch and connected with other people. We are better at reflecting and we are more able to interact socially.

It is also true for those who are underarousal. This is when we have difficulty saying no, setting boundaries, being clear and caring for our space.

What the Survival Instinct and Our Brain Can Do About It

Why it is so hard for us to break out from this traumatic cycle lies with our survival instincts. They have the power to control our actions. These instincts often accomplish this much faster that we realize. This happens when fear is present, but also when our brainstem, the oldest section of the brain, detects imminent danger. This scans our environment throughout the day, looking for any similarity to previous experiences. The brainstem will alert us to danger but there is little we can do.

Because otherwise, most of us would have died by now. When we see a ghost flying towards us we instinctively turn our heads and jump sideways. We don't even know what it is.

The brainstem has the responsibility of regulating the basic bodily functions and ensuring that we survive. The permission of all humans is granted to this oldest brain part, which is vital for our survival. It is not our conscious permission to rule the younger brains for a while and ensure our survival.

When a person has been traumatized, survival scenarios and the survival reaction can often kick in. These survival reactions are sometimes in situations that they don't belong to and may occur too early. This is a serious problem.

The Three Brain Regions

There are three major parts to the brain. The brain stem, approximately 500 million year old, is where instincts and reactions are found. The limbic System was formed 300 million year ago. This system has since influenced our emotions, attachment, and belonging. The neocortex only existed 100,000 years ago. It is here that the mind, which allows us to think abstractly as well as concretely, is found.

These systems have remained partially independent of one another. This may be why we do crazy things. While we know what is healthy for us, we do something else. We know it's not a good idea to panic but we do. This is due to the fact the mind has very limited access both to the emotional and instinctive worlds.

When a Brain Part Takes Over

It's also known as bottom up jacking. This happens when our older brain parts control our behavior. This could last only a few seconds. Sometimes, this can be enough to completely throw someone off course. A friend may approach a woman sitting at a table and put his hand on her leg. This is usually done in a friendly gesture. However, the brainstem is well aware that any type of touching is likely lead to sexual abuse. The woman becomes extremely rigid and quickly dissociates. The woman's frustration and dissociation can lead to severe consequences. This can be used to refer to many situations, reactions, and we rarely realize it.

This is called top-down management. This works only to a limited degree, especially when it concerns areas like fear or trauma.

Talk therapy isn't effective in trauma. Contrary to popular belief, talk therapy can often make trauma worse for those who aren't well-versed in trauma therapy. When they think back to the trauma and speak about it, they often relive it. The result is dissociations or a flood of emotions. Both are not good for your health.

Chapter 7: Overcoming Trauma

T

It is possible to feel safer and more secure after trauma. In the beginning, it's often difficult to create external security.

Peace of Mind and Security

It is more difficult to find inner security. It is not an easy task. This requires patience, stability and maybe professional support such as trauma therapy or counseling.

Take a break, be calm, take the time to rest and relax. Chiefs of operations for disasters, rescue teams, or police officers need to ask this question: How can we find safe areas far away from the disaster site, where the excitement can abate and their consciousness can be re-established? If you are high-aroused, you want to get out of bed and do something. This can often lead to injury or other negative consequences. Reminding people that they don't need to do any of it and that there are others who can help them, can help calm down and reduce the urge to act. Stop those who are in a crisis from jumping up and running.

There are many reasons why it is important to regain your calm. The body's natural healing abilities and recovery processes can only be activated when calm is restored. If the excitement doesn't stop, then you will exhaust your most important resources of strength. A state of exhaustion might eventually occur, and it is not as much related to the traumatizing event as the time following. The engine will keep running at full speed even though there is no destination. You should make use of all tools that can slow down your engine.

Friends, Reassurance, Stability and Helping

It's important that you use any tools that have helped to calm you down. It is important to establish a consistent, routineized daily rhythm in order to help you regain your stability. You can do physical activity, but not too hard, and you should also watch good films. Activities that create stress should be avoided!

It's important to have people or partners that are there for and listen to your needs. Professional support can also be useful if there are no friends or partners.

These are additional tips

Develop helpful habits

Do whatever you can to relax and calm yourself down. Relax, lie down and try to fall asleep. Going for a stroll in familiar surroundings is highly recommended. If your health allows, go for a walk in familiar surroundings. If you're faced with a choice between a movie on TV or your favorite video cassette, go for the latter. The trauma experience can be overwhelming and leaves us with too much unprocessed data. A distraction is more helpful. Do whatever you can to distract yourself.

Try to avoid getting too excited about work. This can create stress. This mistake is all too common. Beelzebub will drive out all the devils. Even if one does manage to distract from trauma, the only thing that will help is exhaustion.

Talk about Trauma

It is important to speak about the trauma you have suffered after it has happened. You must remember to be careful. Some people are unable to stop talking about their trauma. They often become too much for their friends and family, but more so for themselves.

If traumatization took place a long while ago, it is best to talk about it only in a protected setting such as psychotherapy. This is crucial to prevent retraumatization.

Talk to trusted people about these incidents. Be patient and don't get distracted by the immediate situation. Talk slowly and do not rush. They should be able to listen, understand your feelings, and share theirs. They will do this best if they are not personally affected by the same tragic event.

It is important to not let the other person blame you, or lecture you. If this is the norm, it is worth considering whether you have another person who is less affected and more able listen empathically and patiently.

Don't speak to people that you don't trust. Some victims of trauma feel under an obligation to tell everyone their stories. You may feel bored or rejected. Many interlocutors find that they are under their own stress levels and are unwilling or unable to accept the world which is often very threatening. Some are too hurt or are indirectly affected.

The victims feel like they are being victimized and become more isolated from their social networks. If you and your partner can arrange for a small amount of time to discuss the trauma, this can help you stop it from spiraling into a vicious circle. This will help you and your partner. Do not feel obliged to go over the details, which can sometimes be quite painful. It is commonly assumed that this is therapeutically useful.

Instead, the memories can take on a whole new life, and panics are revived. Instead of creating relief, traumatization can be intensified. If your partner is interested in learning more, tell only as much as you can without getting back into the trauma. Ask your partner for their limits. Because trauma is associated with a severe loss of self determination and control over one's own living space, it is important to do all you can in order to bring back that sense of control. It is even more helpful if your surroundings support you in this.

During trauma's shock and impact phases, one must gradually regain a sense of security and safety.

Many who suffer from depression blame themselves for failing, and end up suffering from long-term depression. Here's a quick exercise that may help you to rebuild your self-confidence.

Allow Your Feelings to Be Heard

Even though sudden feelings like anger, sadness, fear, and emptiness may seem unwelcome or inappropriate, it can be healing to allow them. Trauma symptoms can be avoided by allowing them to occur.

Flashback

Flashbacks are flashbacks that look like lightning and can occur when there is a threat. These flashbacks may be much more intense than traditional remembering. Flash backs pose a high risk of re-traumatization so it is important that you interrupt them whenever possible.

To stop flashbacks, move, get up, move around, change rooms, strike yourself with firm and clear strikes, pinch, but most importantly, tell yourself it's a flashback, that the danger has passed, and that you are safe right now.

Be Positive About Your Successes

Please list the ten greatest achievements of your life. Each success should be accompanied by at least five reasons.

Recall your past successes when your life experiences or stressful events are brought up. Take your list of accomplishments with you. If the event is something you've been thinking about for a while now, grab your success list and read it aloud. After some time, the list will no longer be necessary in written form. Take a moment to reflect on your accomplishments, especially if you feel inadequate or afraid.

How the exercise works Then, a paralyzing and depressing mood develops that prevents you from seeing the real world. Recalling past successes can help you break this cycle. Even though the experience was terrible, it is not impossible to overcome. However, for many affected people, it doesn't seem as overwhelming. If you look back at your past successes, the current misery will be confined to your daily life.

This book will give you a number of exercises that can be used to help you cope. They are most effective when each person chooses the exercises that correspond to their individual trauma processing. This requires extensive descriptions of each exercise and a wide range.

Dissociative States

It is normal to feel as though you are slipping out of yourself, sleeping, wrapped in cotton wool, or something similar. This reaction is quite common. It's important to understand how to manage this condition.

The following information can be helpful:

* Understand that the condition is a temporary dissociation. It will end just like any other.

* You must realize that while the ability of dissociation was initially protected, you no longer require it. There are other options.

* To yourself, say phrases like "I'm mature and safe now, I live in a safe area."

* Look down and feel the ground beneath you.

* Keep your hands on a favorite stuffed animal and pay attention to its movements.

* Use cold (e.g., water) to activate your body. Use cold water to wash your hands, arms, face and/or arms.

* Listen soothing music.

* Recognize the differences between now and then. Speak out loudly what the date is today, where are you, and how old are you.

* Find a safe place in your imagination that you can call home.

* Keep your eyes open. Notice the way you breathe in. Breathe in with your eyes closed, focusing more on the exhale.

* Find something that captivates you and activates your senses. For example, read or

view a photograph, listen to music, touch or feel a stone, smell an oil or flower, or consciously taste something salty or spicy.

* Move! Take a walk and shake out.

* Use your hands to create: writing, painting or gardening.

* Take a long, relaxing shower. Focus on your body's touch with the water.

* Have compassion for your self. You are worthy to be kind to your self.

* You should surround yourself with people who are comfortable for you and who don't make you feel uncomfortable.

* Once you're certain, you can say: I am with XX now. Dissociation occurs when I think back to old stories/movies. I am safe now.

* Picture that you are putting everything you hold onto from the past in an safe. You shouldn't let it bother you for the moment.

Keep in mind that this process must be repeated over and over until it becomes automatic and becomes part of your brain. But it will happen one day.

Distancing

It is best to get distance and calm down from traumatizing events in order to prevent any long-term damage.

It is important to remember that you are not just the trauma. To regain your life and body, it is necessary to recognize this.

Not only are we recommending calming exercises but also loving attention to ourselves. The trauma symptoms, signs and dynamics can be used to alleviate fears and facilitate better processing.

Accept Help

Trauma can be described as an event that overwhelms all people. Help is available. There are also professional organizations that offer psychotherapy and counseling.

Trauma Therapy

In many cases, trauma therapy is a good option. These steps are crucial in the therapy:

* Regaining stability.

* Working with the trauma experience.

* Integration (incorporation), of the experience into other areas of life.

Be sure to check that your therapist is familiar with working with traumatized patients before choosing them. Do not be afraid to ask.

Strengthens, not resources

Trauma therapy aims to identify and help people who have been traumatized. All people have the ability to heal themselves. This can be encouraged and supported.

Long-term Trauma

Many women have had to deal with sexual abuse in their childhood. It is not too late! However, the more recent an event is the more complicated the processing. These cases are where professional help is particularly important.

Chapter 8: Recognizing Traumatized People

T

Family members and friends often ask questions about traumatized people's behavior or how to recognize them. You might be asking yourself, "Am I traumatized?" Below are the most frequent symptoms, as well the subtler signs, that can be linked to trauma.

People think of shock trauma almost immediately when they hear the word trauma. Also, classic trauma therapies are used to treat shock trauma. Symptoms such a flashbacks or intrusions are a sign of shock trauma.

However, there is a mix of developmental trauma as well as shock trauma. It is necessary to switch between various interventions. This is where the trauma symptoms are often subtler, making it more difficult to recognize someone who has been traumatized. Over-arousal can be a sign that the nervous system is continually at a very high activity level. Others signs include:

* Insomnia

* Depressions

* Fear

* Concentration difficulties

Tantrums

If there is no one serious experience that triggers a trauma, then it is called a developmental trauma. For example, it can result from long-term trauma or insufficient care and attachment from parents. If such traumatization occurs over a lengthy period of time, it can have devastating effects on our personality. These people are often difficult to recognize and many don't even realize they are suffering from developmental trauma. Affected individuals are often unable to feel their feelings and need and may not be able settle into their bodies.

Traumatized persons: Signs

Post-traumatic Stress Disorder, or PTSD, is not always triggered by a traumatic incident. Others may feel symptoms only after weeks, years or months. These symptoms rarely improve on their own.

These include nightmares, memory problems or stressful memories. Harmless stimuli, such a sound or image, can bring back the trauma experience and inflict intense anxiety. Trauma often manifests in the reliving of the trauma over and again even though it has been long past.

But, the person who is affected does not always experience the entire scenario or see images in his mind's eye. One thing that is consistent is the feeling of helplessness and fear experienced by the affected individual. Other than heart palpitations or physical stress, it is possible to experience other symptoms such as anxiety and panic attacks. An example of a trauma experience is insomnia, jumpiness or difficulty concentrating.

Many people affected try to avoid situations that may remind them of such an experience. This can include avoiding these places and suppressing thoughts about what is happening. Other symptoms include depression, emotional exhaustion, and withdrawal from social situations. Some people react to depressive moods and shame or guilt.

PTSD can cause pain and addiction. OCD, depression, anxiety disorders and obsessive/compulsive disorder are all possible. Children may experience a temporary regression in their developmental process. Some suffer from stomach ache and headaches. How can one be identified?

Behavior of traumatized persons

People with shock trauma can be easily identified in everyday life by the way they talk about the event. A shock trauma is something that people with it cannot talk about. They may be overwhelmed by the memory, or they may dissociate as they tell the story. But there are some clues that can indicate shock trauma.

* It appears as if the events just happened.

* We listen but feel uncomfortable listening.

* You are attracted to the traumatic pull.

* A flattened voice can be a sign that someone is not using modulation.

* Lack of emotion - There is little emotion to be seen in the face or the faces of others.

* People tell the story in an unprofessional way. In an inappropriate setting or with inappropriate facial expressions, such as laughter.

* Those who are affected feel overwhelmed by emotions and have difficulty containing them.

It is the event that one cannot identify as traumatization, and this time it is! Trauma lies in your nervous system, which is the human response to the event. It is unknown why some events can be traumatizing or not for others.

It is believed to be connected to the following factors.

* The ability for self-regulation.

* Believe.

* To participate in a group.

* Resources in Life

* Resource information at the event.

This resistance is also known as resilience.

Recognizing a Traumatization is not a substitute for the diagnosis

Perhaps you already know the meaning of trauma, and are able to recognize people who have been traumatized. The self-diagnosis of trauma does not replace the diagnosis made by a qualified therapist. Only by carefully examining the patient can traumata be identified.

Recognizing that traumatization can be the source of one's own symptoms and suffering can feel like finding the right key to oneself. You can then find the right path to help you cope with trauma therapy.

How to Help Traumatized Individuals

A special technique is used to gently and effectively treat trauma symptoms during intensive therapy. This treatment lasts for three days. The best thing about this method is that it does not take long or expensive therapy.

Both outpatient and inpatient therapies can identify the problem and provide treatment. In rare cases, medication is not necessary. If needed, you can relieve symptoms with the help of mental blocks.

The first task is to find the traumatic events in your subconscious. For talk therapy to work, the patient must clearly recognize what is causing the mental injury. Sometimes it is necessary for the patient's memory to contain the traumatic event.

People who have been traumatized by disturbing events can benefit from therapy. There are several building blocks to support their treatment. It is common to use pharmacotherapy as well as psychotherapy in the treatment of trauma. Different treatment options are available depending on the severity of the trauma.

Psychoeducation is another useful option. It enables the patients to be informed about their condition and the clinical picture. Ergotherapy, sociotherapy, and relaxation are all possible additional therapeutic methods.

Different effects can result from the experience. The therapy is tailored to the individual's preferences and the impairments caused. Based on severity and type, support methods may be suggested.

Chapter 9: Combating Ptsd

P

TSD is the acronym of Post-Traumatic Stress Disorder. Many people also use the acronym PTSD to signify Post-Traumatic Stress Syndrome Disorder. Trauma-related disorder, another term for PTSD, is also used. These terms are used to describe intense psychological reactions that can be attributed to extremely stressful life events. These reactions are marked by a repeated reliving trauma, emotional and/or social withdrawal, as well as nervous and physical excitement.

What is PTSD and how can it be treated?

Post-traumatic stress disorder (PTSD), is a group that includes adjustment and stress disorders. These are psychological reactions that can be clearly traced back at extremely stressful life events.

Trauma combined with PTSD can feel like a shopping bag, or a suitcase you leave in the hallway. It is like a bag you keep falling on until you finally get rid of it. The brain switches off certain parts during trauma to prevent the experience from being stored in a time-stamped format. These events can be found behind every door. We experience them as though they are happening right now. It can have a major impact on the lives and well-being of people with post-traumatic Stress Disorder.

How does PTSD develop

Trauma Disorder, also known as Post-Traumatic Trauma Disorder (PTSD), can be referred too. Now, what exactly is trauma? A trauma experience is any experience that makes someone feel helpless, powerless, and out-of-control. This can happen from a serious accident to abuse of power, sexual abuse or rape, as well as an experience of war. Being excluded from a group (bullying), making a condescending remark at inappropriate times, or witnessing a frightening event can all trigger these feelings. In these situations, certain brain regions are activated: the ones required for an automatic reaction, known as fight, flight, and freeze reflexes.

But, some parts are also turned off, including those who are responsible to save in the biographical library. Stimuli of similarity are now able to evoke these memories. The feeling that it was all gone is gone if the experience is not archived. The experience is recreated and experienced in all its intensity. This causes the person to experience the same stress over and over again as the original. The language center is also turned off, so that it's impossible to describe what happened. The person feels the intensity of the experience again. This causes the person to experience the same stress over and over again as before.

Van der Kolk's most recent findings suggest that trauma healing requires a technique that follows:

* Calm activated brain areas.

* Activate the brain regions that are currently off.

This is what TBT, which combines tapping and acupressure with elements of neuro-linguistic program (NLP), does.

Symptoms of Post Traumatic Stress Disorder

The person who suffers from post-traumatic stress disorder may experience a loss of self-confidence and security. This can happen right away after the trauma or it may occur weeks, months, and even years later. An example of this is when the victim remembers the traumatizing experience from childhood but has now lost the ability to fully recall it.

Symptoms of PTSD include:

* Intrusive memories: Recurrent experiences of the traumatic event in imagination (flashback), or as a dream.

* Avoiding similar situations

* Emotional withdrawal and social withdrawal

* Nervous or physical overexcitement.

More precisely, the symptoms associated with PTSD can be broken down into:

* A vegetative hyperexcitement is an overexcited state of alertness, irritability, jumpiness and sleep disturbances.

* Avoidance behavior. Victims will avoid situations, people, places, or activities that might trigger memories of the trauma. A victim who has survived a plane wreckage will not only not fly again but will also avoid any situations that could trigger memories. Some people with PTSD experience extreme emotional isolation, such as inner apathy or indifference.

* A re-experiencing the trauma: repeated intrusive memory (intrusion), flashbacks and nightmares. Flashbacks are typically triggered with a trigger (also called a key stimuli). This can be a loud bang or special voice.

In a fraction, the person is brought back to life their past trauma (e.g. A war or rape, the person is brought back to that trauma with all their emotions, fears, and painful feelings. It is a recollection, but the subject feels that he is in the same place as before. He is again able to experience the horror. During flashbacks, he does not see the real environment and does no respond to being spoken.

Not only is it exhausting, but repeated trauma can also cause suffering and re-traumatize. These three symptoms are called the symptom triad.

Many are affected by the loss of their worldview that people are generally safe from danger and are not helpless. They have a hard time trusting people and are very cautious. Some people feel shame and may even feel self-loathing.

Phenomenas Of Intrusion (Reliving).

* The painful memories of the trauma keep coming back to haunt the person.

* Dreams and nightmares about the stressful events.

* Spontaneous acting, feeling and thinking as during the traumatic incident (flashbacks).

* Emotional disturbances caused by trauma (peoples and places, words, objects or activities).).

* Physical reactions to something that is traumatizing.

Cognition and mood change

* Memory gaps related to the traumatic experience.

* Feeling of being separate from oneself and watching oneself as if outside.

* Persistent, repetitive experiences of unreality or distorted, alien, dreamlike.

* Negative selfimage and worldview

* Persistent feelings such as deep despair, fear or panic, anger and guilt.

* Feelings or guilt towards others and oneself.

* A persistent inability to see anything good in life.

Changes to Excitability and Responsiveness

Hypervigilance refers to excessive vigilance of the sufferer who constantly checks the environment for signs that are reminiscent or the trauma.

* Excessive Startle Reactions

* Difficulty concentrating.

* Sleep disorders.

* Self-aggressive behaviors.

International Classification of Diseases - ICD-10 lists PTSD as one of the mental disorders.

A person who has suffered trauma often feels emotionally deadened. This can include a feeling of indifference to other people and an inability to accept the environment. The trauma fear can often lead to the person avoiding certain situations and cues that might trigger memories.

Causes of Post Traumatic Stress Disorder

Common triggers for PTSD are:

* War operations and terrorist attacks; political imprisonment.

* A violent crime committed by someone such as robbery (or rape), kidnapping, or torture.

* A serious accident.

* Disasters (fires and avalanches, earthquakes or a flood disaster like a tsunami), but also explosions or a crash of a plane, train, or other vehicle.

* A life-threatening diagnosis (e.g., cancer, heart condition) or a medical emergency that needs to be treated in an intensive care unit.

Traumatic experiences can also occur in relationships, as an example is domestic violence. Infidelity is a situation where the trust is shattered and the victim can feel angry, fearful, self-doubt, helplessness, and other symptoms. But it's not post-traumatic stress disorder. The betrayer doesn't fear for the future and doesn't have flashbacks or reliving trauma.

Prognosis & Course in PTSD

Post-traumatic Stress Disorder is a complex clinical picture. The course of the condition varies from one patient to another. The duration, severity, and frequency of PTSD (complex PTSD), as well as the individual resilience of the affected person will all affect the time it takes for PTSD healing to occur. Some people have greater mental resilience, which psychologists call resilience. Others have greater vulnerability.

Some of the victims also feel symptoms immediately after trauma. However, some others experience symptoms for months or years, while others only have a few symptoms.

Complex post-traumatic stress disorder is generally treatable. Studies have shown that PTSD symptoms usually improve within a year for about a third to a quarter of the people affected. Two-thirds (33%) of patients with PTSD will experience it for the rest of their lives. 80 percent of the patients affected will also experience other mental disorders such as depression and anxiety.

This can cause a loss of quality of life. As a result, people affected may have difficulty in their relationships, friendships, or at work. This can lead to divorce, job losses, financial hardship, social isolation, or even social isolation. Post-traumatic stress disorder must be treated promptly.

Impact of PTSD On the Lives of Those Affected

Rehana's story of how a traumatic experience can impact a person's ability to live a normal life shows this. After working with New Zealand's recidivists, she discovered that they were all traumatized. She used a variety of techniques to treat trauma, and eventually developed her own method. It proved to be very effective. None of the offenders she treated suffered from relapse. However, we can conclude that these individuals were suffering from PTSD (post-traumatic Stress Disorder) or traumatic afflictions.

A Trauma disorder is actually a survival strategy for nature

Why is each experience processed differently? If the trauma memories cause only restlessness, insomnia and panic attacks, then what is the point? Is there a reason or a misstep by nature?

This is because trauma processing takes place within the reptilian's brain. This is the brain our ancestors and I have shared for many years - millions of year. For an animal to escape from a dangerous situation it must only perceive signs that it might be in. All symptoms of PTSD can increase the likelihood of survival in situations in which the person is endangered. Particularly if victim is a mouse, lizard or gazelle.

Humans are endowed with our ability to think and use our minds to evaluate dangers. We don't need to fight for our survival every day.

The reptilian brain, however, doesn't know all this. It tries to protect itself from dangers that don't exist. It doesn't mean that we have to constantly fight for survival. The reptilian brain, however, doesn't know all this so it protects us from any dangers that aren't there.

Diagnosis and Treatment of PTSD

Post-Traumatic Syndrome Disorder (PTSD), a mental disorder, is one example. It is a member of the group of adjustment disorders and stress disorders. These include acute stress reactions as well as adjustment disorders. The acute stress response occurs within minutes of the event and lasts approximately 2-3 days. It is often called a nervous breakdown.

It can cause numbness, panic, anxiety, sweating and tremors as well as restlessness, overactivity, amnesia, depression symptoms and social withdrawal. It is most common to resolve without therapy. However, it may progress to post-traumatic Stress Disorder.

An adjustment disorder arises from a life change, e.g. It can occur in the case of the death, or cultural shock. This is characterised by anxiety, depressed mood, worry, and panic. It starts within 4 weeks after the change in lifestyle. However it doesn't last for more that 6 months.

Post-Traumatic Stress Disorder is clearly a result from a traumatic incident (post-traumatic methods after trauma). The severity of symptoms will depend on how severe one is, what the victim was exposed to, their proximity and the length of time. If the symptoms last more then a month, it is considered PTSD. Before diagnosing PTSD, an examination should rule out other causes.

A doctor or psychologist will conduct a thorough conversation about the patient's psychological and physical symptoms, as well as his or her medical history (anamnesis). He or she will also ask about any risk factors that could lead to PTSD (e.g. The patient's family and friends support, if they had any mental illness or a family history, as well as whether or not they were able to provide much help after the trauma.

According to the psychiatric rating system, post-traumatic Stress Disorder is when a person has experienced trauma and experiences intrusions or avoidance behavior. The symptoms should have been present for at most one month and seriously affect the patient's life quality.

For a more specific diagnosis, there are several tests. The expert usually uses scientifically standardized questionnaires, an example of which is the CAPS questionnaire (Clinician-Administered PTSD Scale). The therapist will ask the patient approximately 20 questions about their symptoms. These include when they started, how long they last, what frequency they are, and how severe they are. The therapist might ask the patient, for example, whether there have been instances in the past month when you felt or acted suddenly as if your trauma was actually happening again. Are you having any reactions to touching or touching other people? What was the traumatizing event? Which situations trigger such reactions?

PTSD sufferers are often very insecure and have difficulty talking openly about their problems. They are often unable to do this unless they trust the therapist.

This is crucial for the therapist to understand the increased security requirements of PTSD patients. He or she should, for example, maintain a sufficient distance from the patient, allow the door to open, and remove any triggers from their conversation.

If the patient is suffering from other mental disorders, it should be taken into consideration when determining a diagnosis. Post-traumatic Stress Disorder is rarely a single condition. It often occurs in conjunction with depression and/or addiction. Additionally, anxiety disorders are common. It may be necessary to treat an addiction in an addiction clinic.

The Acute stress reaction is the first response to a stressful event.

People who have experienced an emotionally extreme situation such as a sudden dismissal, separation or accident often exhibit strong stress symptoms. This includes an accelerated heartbeat and head pressure. They also may experience nauseousness, nausea, vomiting, and a change in their behavior. The symptoms of stress include restlessness and irritability as well as disorientation (the feeling that one is watching the serious events unfold).

This is what psychologists call the acute stress reaction. It often occurs right after an event and usually subsides within hours, days or a minimum of a month.

Even in cases where trauma is involved, the individual suffering from it will feel the effects of an acute stress response. If it persists, it could lead to a mental disorder called post-traumatic Stress Disorder.

Trouble accepting a life-changing event: The Adjustment Disorder

Some people find it difficult to adjust to a change in their life. A person may have an adjustment disorder if they refuse to accept the split that their partner has decided on. They might also believe that everything will be just fine for the next few months even though there is no evidence of it. This is often due to strong fears. Depression can also be a result.

Adjustment Disorders and PTSD

Adjustment disorder means that a person has difficulty accepting a change in their situation. A person suffering from post-traumatic Stress Disorder (or over-arousal) experiences the trauma in flashbacks, dreams, or in constant alertness.